# Brachial Plexus Injury - New Techniques and Ideas

*Edited by Jörg Bahm*

Published in London, United Kingdom

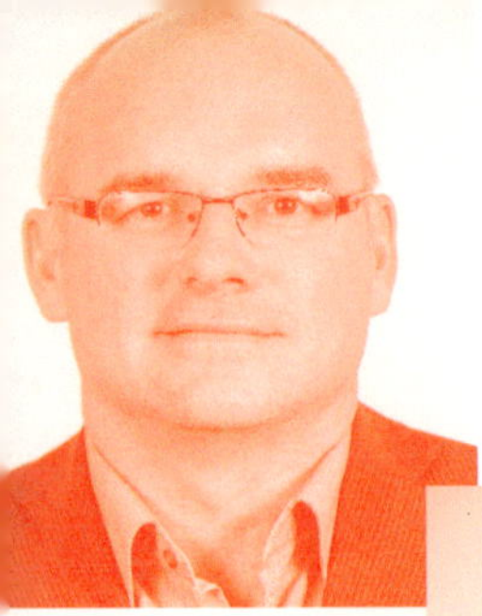
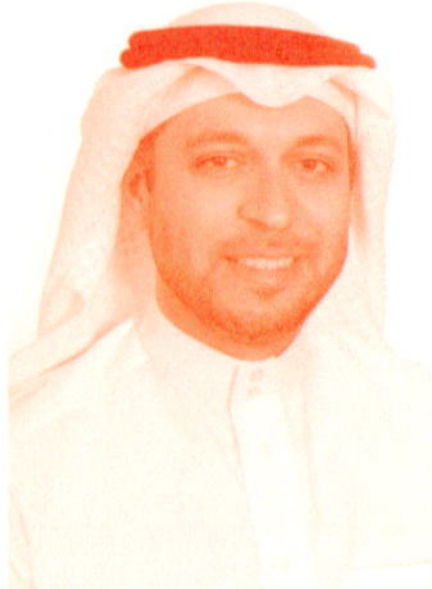
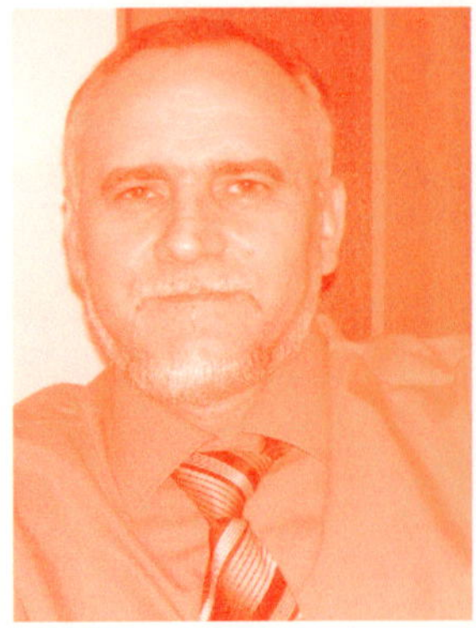
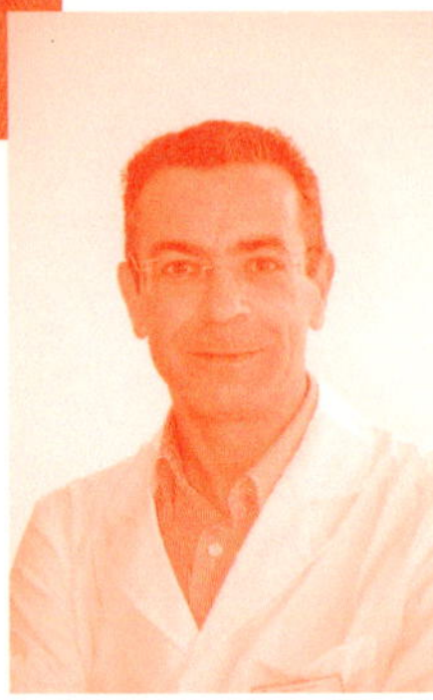
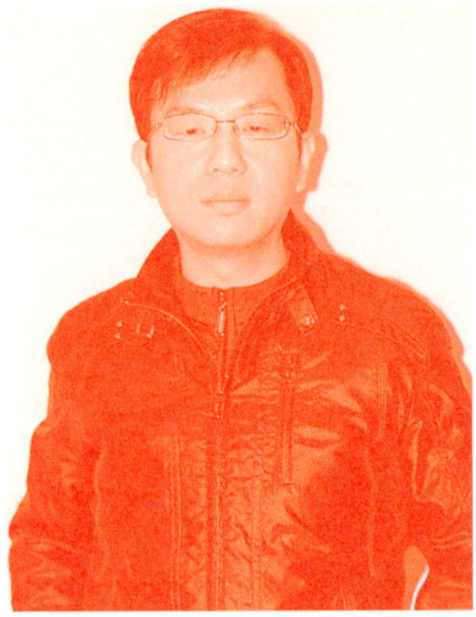
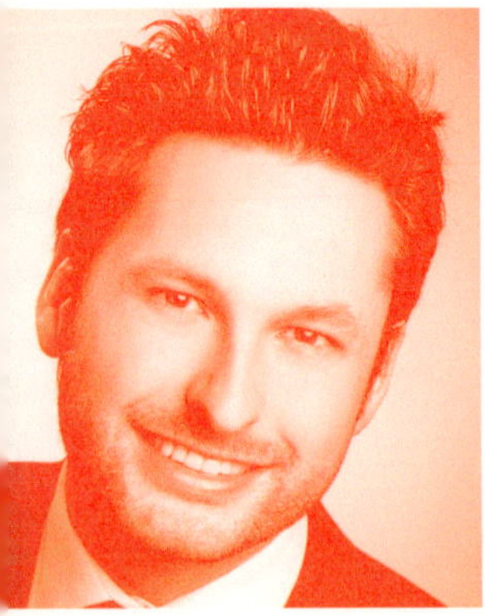
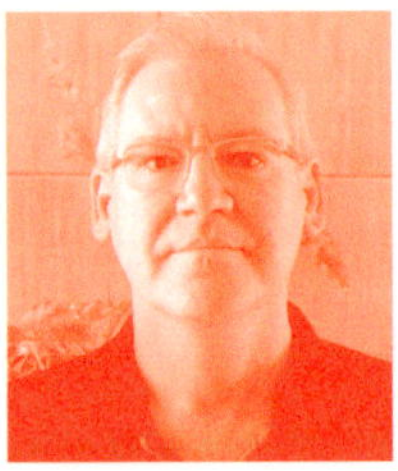

IntechOpen

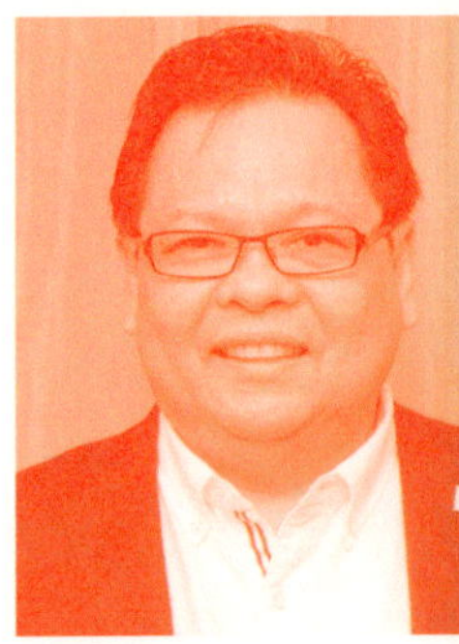
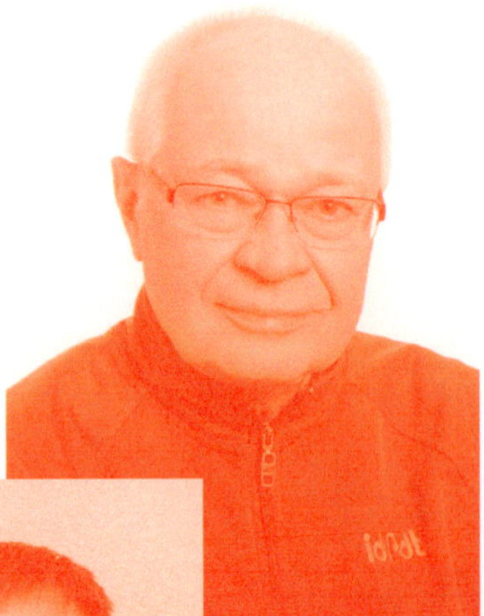
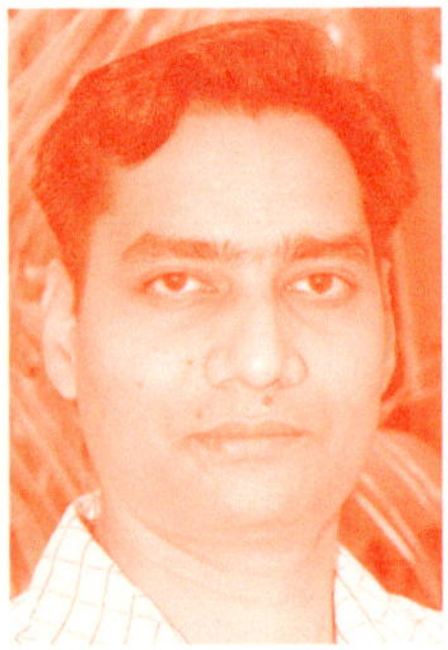
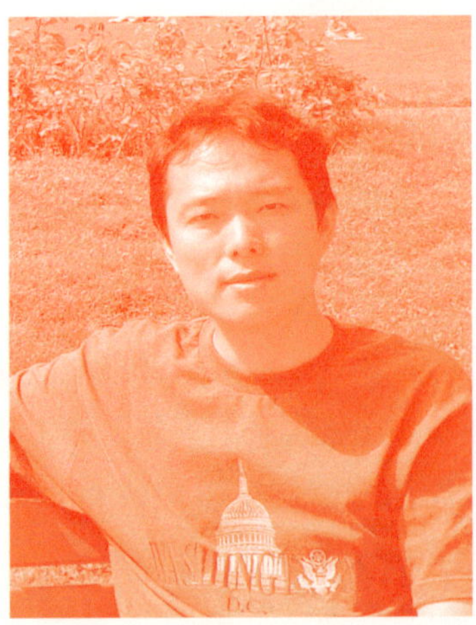
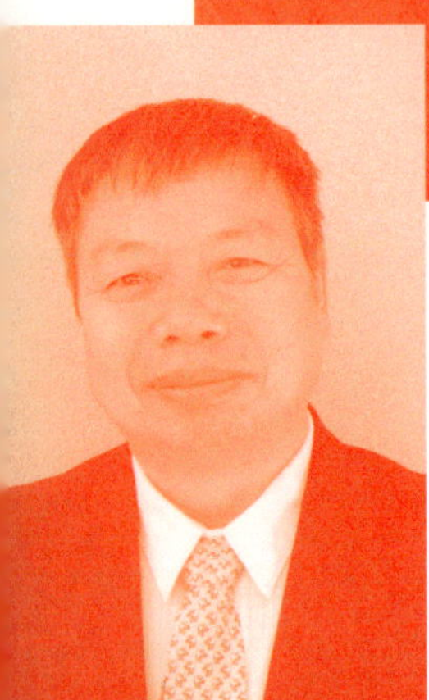
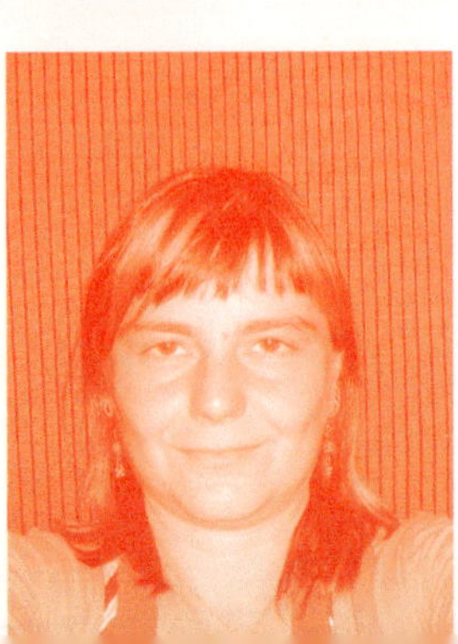

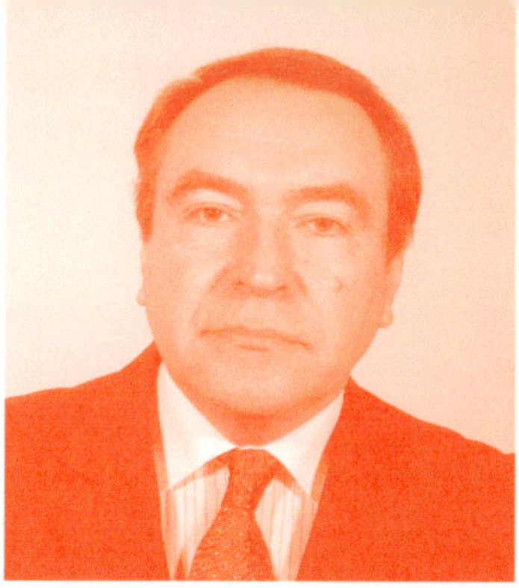
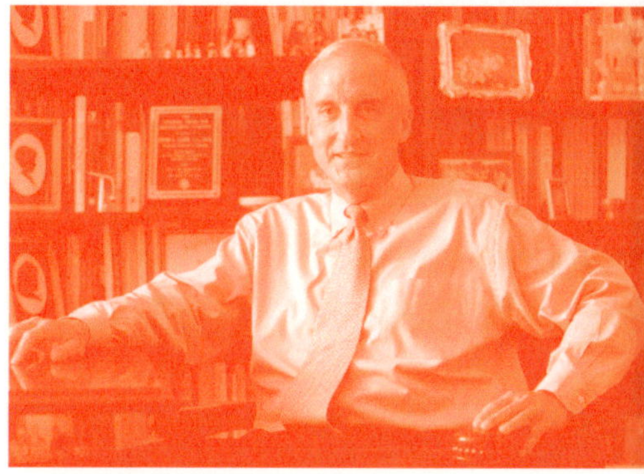
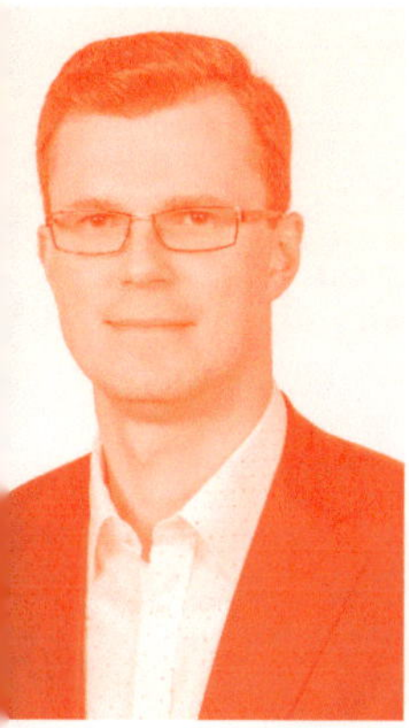
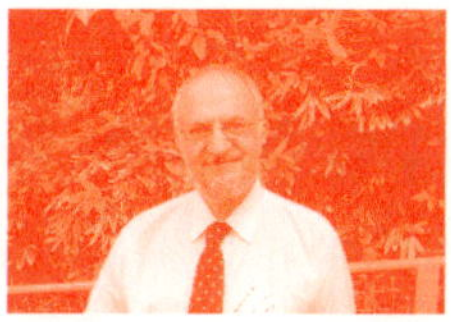
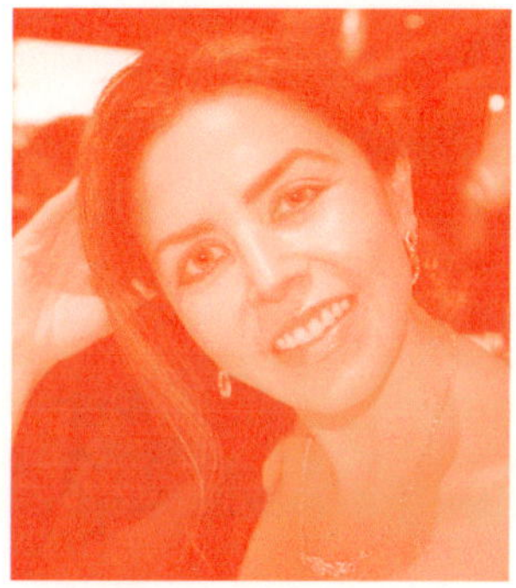

*Supporting open minds since 2005*

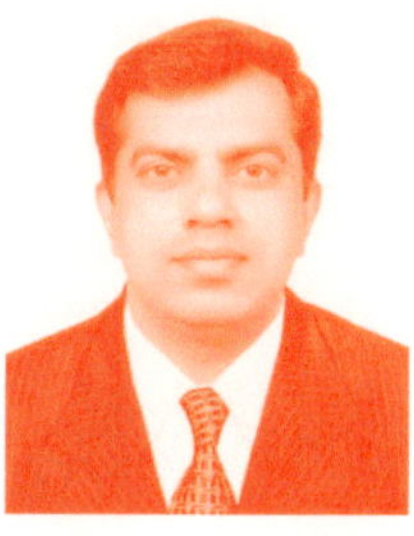
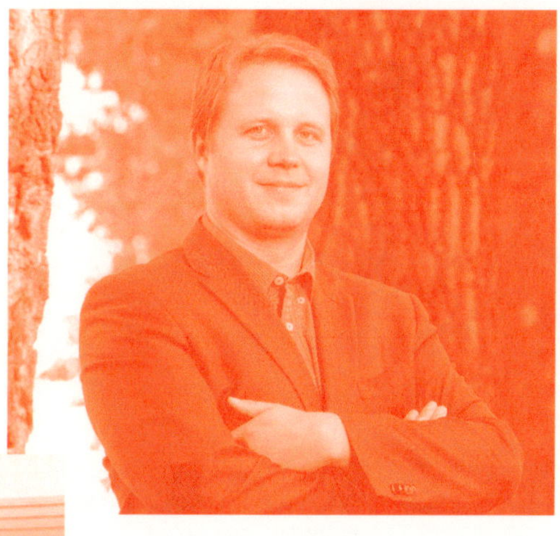
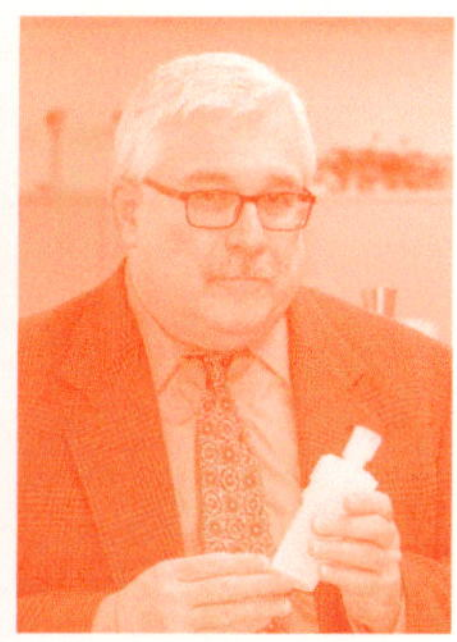
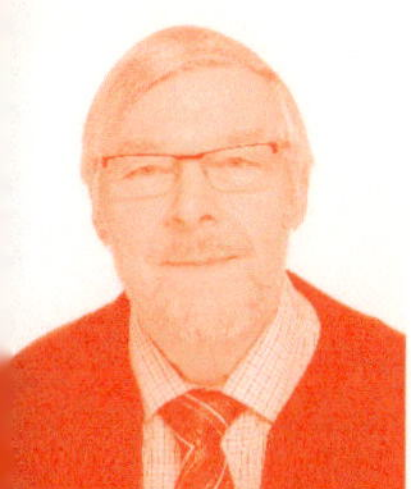
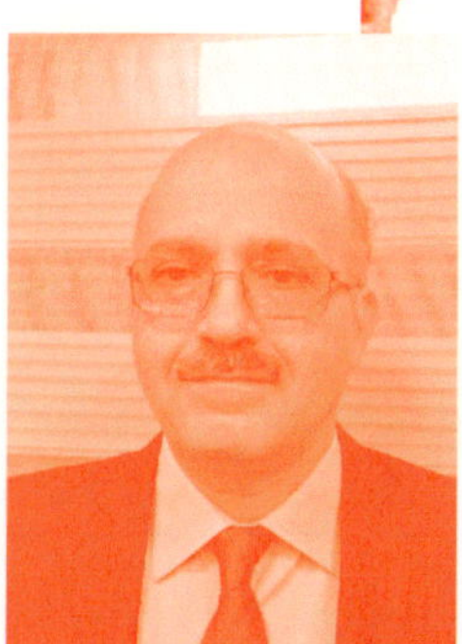
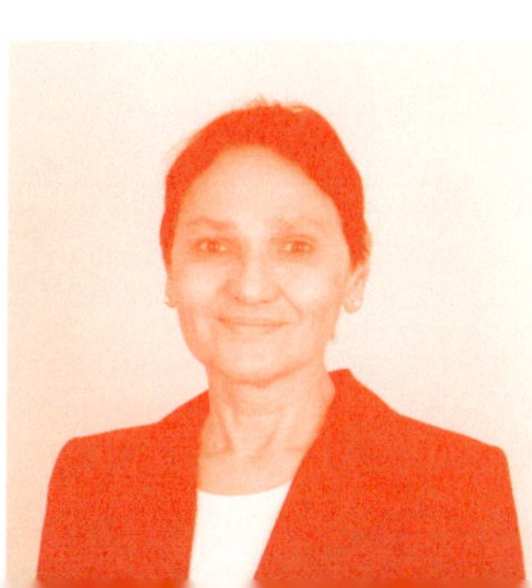
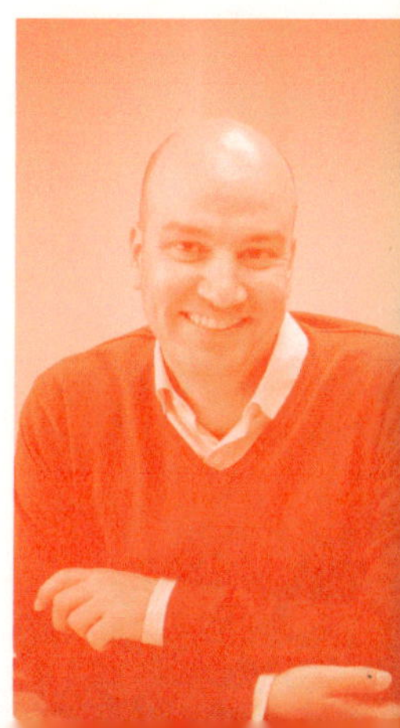

Brachial Plexus Injury - New Techniques and Ideas
http://dx.doi.org/10.5772/intechopen.94695
Edited by Jörg Bahm

Contributors
Joseph M. Rosen, Jennifer Hong, Julien Klaudt-Moreau, Allison Podsednik, Vincent R. Hentz, Nora F. Dengler, Jennifer Reinsch, Anna Zdunczyk, Tarik Alp Sargut, Maren Denker, Melina Engelhardt, Peter Vajkoczy, Thomas Picht, Jean-Noel Goubier, Frédéric Teboul, Camille Echalier, Elodie Dubois, Grainne Bourke, Mikael Wiberg, Lev Novikov, Andrew Hart, Teodor Stamate, Dan Cristian Moraru, Ahmet Emrah Açan, Ertuğrul Şahin, Alexander A. Gatskiy, Ihor B. Tretyak, Lin Yang, Jia He, YaXuan Li, MengNan Jiang, Qianling Zhang, Aleksandra McGrath, Alice Chu, Shivani Gupta, Jasmine Mahajan, Nivetha Srinivasan, Amy Song, Jörg Bahm



First published in London, United Kingdom, 2022 by IntechOpen
IntechOpen is the global imprint of INTECHOPEN LIMITED, registered in England and Wales, registration number: 11086078, 5 Princes Gate Court, London, SW7 2QJ, United Kingdom
Printed in Croatia

British Library Cataloguing-in-Publication Data
A catalogue record for this book is available from the British Library

Additional hard and PDF copies can be obtained from orders@intechopen.com

Brachial Plexus Injury - New Techniques and Ideas
Edited by Jörg Bahm
p. cm.
Print ISBN 978-1-83969-686-2
Online ISBN 978-1-83969-687-9
eBook (PDF) ISBN 978-1-83969-688-6

For EU product safety concerns:
IN TECH d.o.o., Prolaz Marije Krucifikse Kozulić 3, 51000 Rijeka, Croatia, info@intechopen.com or visit our website at intechopen.com.

# Meet the editor

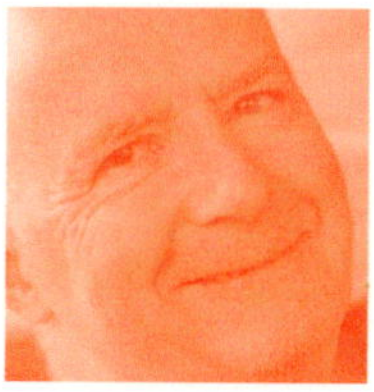

Jörg Bahm obtained an MD in 1987 and a Ph.D. from Université libre de Bruxelles (ULB), Brussels, Belgium in 2011. As a general, plastic, and hand surgeon, Dr. Bahm worked for five years at University Hospital Aachen, Germany. Since 1994, he has focused on brachial plexus surgery. He has been a chief surgeon in the Reconstructive Microsurgery Unit of the Franziskushospital, Aachen, Germany since 2000. In 2020, this unit was transferred into the Aachen University Hospital as the Division for Plexus Surgery within the Department for Plastic, Hand and Burn Surgery. Since 2003, Dr. Bahm has been a consultant for peripheral nerves in the Orthopaedic Department, Erasme University Hospital, Brussels, Belgium. He is an active member of the German (DGH) and Belgian (BHG) Hand Surgery Society and of the German Plastic Surgery Society (DGPRÄC). He is a member of the Narakas club for brachial plexus surgery and editor of the online *Journal of Brachial Plexus and Peripheral Nerve Injury*. He has written more than 50 scientific papers and presented at more than 200 congresses. Dr. Bahm was president of the BHG in 2012 and 2013 and congress president of the FESSH Hand Surgery congress 2012 in Antwerp, Belgium. His specific interests are peripheral nerve surgery and microsurgical reconstruction of the upper limb.

# Contents

# Preface

Brachial plexus surgery remains an innovating field within functional reconstructive surgery, especially due to the expanding use of nerve transfers in the last twenty years.

Dealing with patients suffering from a brachial plexus or related lesion, either obstetrical or traumatic, infection or tumor, nerve compression or rupture, is a permanent challenge. Better techniques in nerve transfers and their use for tetra- or paraplegia, spasticity, or arthrogryposis are examples of advancements in the field.

Our wish is that this book allows further insight and discussion, stimulates experts and newcomers, and adds to our global knowledge of brachial plexus injury and treatment.

I wish to thank the staff at IntechOpen, particularly Project Manager Karmen Đaleta, for their assistance throughout the publication process.

**Jörg Bahm**
Division of Plexus Surgery,
Department for Plastic,
Hand and Burn Surgery,
RWTH University Hospital,
Aachen, Germany

Section 1

# Introduction

Chapter 1

# Introductory Chapter: Treatment of Brachial Plexus Lesions - A New Transdisciplinary Approach

*Jörg Bahm*

## 1. Introduction

A *discipline* is defined as a group of experts sharing the same body of knowledge.

There are several medical and also surgical and other disciplines involved in peripheral nerve reconstruction, such as neuro-, plastic, orthopaedic or hand surgeons, physio- and occupational therapists, neuropathologists, and bio-engineers.

The neurosurgeon is considered an expert in surgical treatment of pathologies within the central and peripheral nervous system and has particular knowledge in nerve anatomy, the physiology of nerve de- and regeneration, direct nerve repair techniques, microsurgery.

The orthopedic surgeon has specialized in bones and joints static and dynamic corrections and functional surgery of the lower limb, whereas the plastic surgeon deals with soft tissue and microsurgery and performs muscle and tendon transfers as well as small vessel and nerve microsurgery—hand and peripheral nerve surgery.

These attributions are of course country/continent dependent.

Giving an image to possible interactions between disciplines, a *multidisciplinary* approach assembles several disciplines in parallel, like several fruits placed in a basket. The routine interaction is *interdisciplinary*, like fruit pieces in a fruit salad. A *transdisciplinary* approach raises totally new issues, like in the creation of a smoothie.

## 2. The concept of transdisciplinarity

Already in 1970, Jean Piaget stated that " a child is not a small adult."

In 1996, the French-Romanian physicist Basarab Nicolescu published a "manifest" about transdisciplinarity, where he developed it as a strong concept, but open and tolerant, transgressing frontiers between disciplines. He cited quantic physics, where the quantum (M. Planck: discontinuity of energy) may be seen as a particle or wave. There is also the time–space indeterminism (Heisenberg) and thus different levels of reality. Facing complex issues, one observes multiplication of disciplines.

Stephane Lupasco, a French-Romanian philosopher, introduced the " **included third**": Extending the concept of " A and non A" known in *classic* physics with the addition of a third status (being neither A nor " non A") in *quantic* physics.

Transdisciplinary approaches are actually seen in **science**, like physics; in **medicine**, like for general practitioners [1], in psychiatry-psychoanalysis, for example, in the treatment of psychopathy [2], emergency care of polytraumatized [3], oncology [4], and geriatrics [5].

It has to be distinguished from **translational** medicine (*"from bench to bed"*).

We also find it in **nursing**, overall in palliative care [6] and even **politics**—like in Bhutan, the concept of "gross national happiness."

## 3. Examples in reconstructive brachial plexus surgery

1. *think beyond the nerve repair one to one*

Some target nerves are more important than others for functional recovery. In obstetric brachial plexus palsy, the re-innervation of the suprascapular nerve is mandatory for a dynamic rotational equilibrium of the glenohumeral joint, a condition allowing congruent development of the joint partners and preventing dysplasia [7]. Thus, in specific conditions, this nerve must be targeted separately by a good motor donor nerve, like the distal/caudal branch of the spinal accessory nerve [8].

2. *think beyond the nerve alone: transfers of one or two motor intercostal nerves onto the thoracodorsalis and thoracicus longus nerve allow to re-innervate during primary surgery such major target muscles than the latissimus dorsi (transferable for elbow flexion or extension later on if needed) and the serratus anterior (stabilizing the scapula, mandatory in case of a later glenohumeral arthrodesis in adult patients).*

3. *think global: Glenohumeral arthrodesis may be a late option to recreate a stable, and basically mobile shoulder.*

4. *think life quality: consider the specific treatment of neuropathic pain, the rare indications for amputation of a flail limb.*

5. *integrate all aspects and tissues in your strategy, beyond your own basic specialty/ discipline!*


## Author details

Jörg Bahm
Division of Plexus Surgery, Department for Plastic, Hand and Burn Surgery, RWTH University Hospital, Aachen, Germany

*Address all correspondence to: jorg.bahm@belgacom.net

## References

[1] Lynch JM, Dowrick C, Meredith P, McGregor SLT, van Driel M. Transdisciplinary Generalism: Naming the epistemology and philosophy of the generalist. Journal of Evaluation in Clinical Practice. 2021;**27**(3):638-647. DOI: 10.1111/jep.13446. [Epub 2020 September 16]

[2] Jean-Pierre C. From pluridisciplinarity to transdisciplinarity. Cliniques. 2012;**No 3**:96-114. DOI: 10.3917/clini.003.0096. URL. Available from: https://www.cairn-int.info/journal-cliniques-2012-1-page-96.htm

[3] Lapierre A, Gauvin-Lepage J, Lefebvre H. La collaboration interprofessionnelle lors de la prise en charge d'un polytraumatisé aux urgences : Une revue de la littérature [Interprofessional collaboration in the management of a polytrauma at the emergency department : a literature review.]. Recherche en Soins Infirmiers. 2017;**129**:73-88. French. DOI: 10.3917/rsi.129.0073

[4] Fernandes I, Rueff MC, Portela S. Transdisciplinarity in strategic decisions for oncological treatments. Medicine and Law. 2015;**34**(1):645-659

[5] Sargent L, Slattum P, Brooks M, Gendron T, Mackiewicz M, Diallo A, et al. iCubed health and wellness in aging transdisciplinary core. Bringing transdisciplinary aging research from theory to practice. Gerontologist. 2020:gnaa214. DOI: 10.1093/geront/gnaa214. Epub ahead of print

[6] Michel P. Transdisciplinarity: A prerequisite for palliative care practice. Revue Internationale de Soins Palliatifs. 2007;**22**:19-22. DOI: 10.3917/inka.071.0019. URL https://www.cairn-int.info/journal-infokara-2007-1-page-19.htm

[7] Nicolescu B. Manifesto of Transdisciplinarity. Albany- State University of New York Press; 2002

[8] Nicolescu B. Stéphane Lupasco et le tiers inclus. Revue de Synthèse. 2005; **126**:431-441

Section 2

# Surgical Techniques

Chapter 2

# Nerve Transfers for Restoring Elbow Flexion in Brachial Plexus Palsy

*Teodor Stamate and Dan Cristian Moraru*

## Abstract

Nerve transfers (NT) consist in sectioning a donor nerve and connecting it to the distal stump of a recipient unrepairable nerve. For elbow flexion restoration in brachial plexus palsy (BPP) we used different NT: 1) GF motor Ulnar Nerve to Biceps nerve (Oberlin technique), 2) Double fascicular median/ulnar to biceps/brachialis nerve transfer (Mackinnon), 3) InterCostal Nerves (ICN) to MCN (+/− nerve graft), 4) Medial Pectoral Nerve (MPN) to MCN, 5) ThoracoDorsal Nerve (TDN) to MCN, 6) Spinal Accessory Nerve (SAN) to MCN transfer, 7) Phrenic Nerve (PhN) to MCN, 8) Cervical Plexus C3-C4 to MCN and 9) Contralateral C7 (CC7). I want to present my personal experience using the phrenic nerve (PhN), the intercostal nerves (ICN) and Oberlin's technique. The aim of this retrospective study is to evaluate the results of this procedure in BPP. NT is an important goal in BPP. ICN transfer into the nerve of biceps for elbow flexion recovery is a reliable procedure in BPP. ICN transfer for triceps offers a positive alternative (Carroll transposition). Oberlin technique is simple and offers better results in a shorter amount of time and is an effective and safe option.

**Keywords:** brachial plexus, nerve transfer, elbow flexion

## 1. Introduction

A complete functional recovery is the ultimate goal in the treatment of brachial plexus injury. However, in most of our patients, this goal cannot be achieved due to the severity of the injuries and the restriction of donor nerves.

The priorities of functional reconstruction in brachial plexus injury have been set as follows [1], in order: 1) elbow flexion; 2) shoulder abduction; 3) wrist and finger flexion and sensation in the median nerve distribution; 4) wrist and finger extension; 5) intrinsic muscle function.

## 2. Nerve transfers

**Nerve transfers for elbow flexion are:**

1. Motor fascicular groups (FG) Ulnar Nerve to Biceps nerve (Oberlin technique)
2. Double fascicular median/ulnar to biceps/brachialis nerve transfer (Mackinnon)

3. InterCostal Nerves (ICN) to Musculocutaneous nerve (MCN) (+/− nerve graft)

4. Medial Pectoral Nerve (MPN) to MCN

5. Thoraco Dorsal Nerve (TDN) to MCN

6. Spinal Accessory Nerve (SAN) to MCN transfer

7. Phrenic Nerve (PhN) to MCN

8. Cervical Plexus C3-C4 to MCN

9. Contralateral C7 (CC7)

### 2.1 Motor FG ulnar nerve to biceps nerve (Oberlin technique)

In 1990 – Oberlin proposed the transfer of motor FG's from the ulnar nerve to the biceps branch of the MCN without an intervening nerve graft; the motor branch from the musculocutaneous nerve to the biceps muscle and the ulnar nerve were found at the midarm level [2]. After performing a 2–3 cm longitudinal epineurotomy in the ulnar nerve, one or two fascicles are found and sutured end to end to the branch of the nerve to the biceps by 3 or 4 stitches of 10–0 nylon. 90% of the patients achieve better than MRC grade 4 elbow flexion with the Oberlin technique [3]. Intraoperative electrostimulation to identify motor FG's of the ulnar nerve is mandatory [4]. The contraindications for Oberlin technique are: lesion of C7-C8-T1 (electromyography (EMG) before surgery on the donor nerve – ulnar nerve – is mandatory); long delay between injury and surgery (**Figure 1**) [5].

### 2.2 Mackinnon technique

In 2005, MacKinnon proposed to modify the original Oberlin procedure to include reinnervation of the brachialis branch of the MCN using the motor FG's of the median nerve [6]. The ideal median nerve donor fascicle contains nerves to the flexor digitorum superficialis (FDS) and flexor carpi radialis (FCR) and intraoperative electrostimulation for motor fascicle of median nerve causes wrist flexion [7]. Several reports have been published comparing single and dual reinnervation, and despite the intuitive logic that more is better, the most recent prospective randomized trial did not demonstrate any difference in objective outcomes between the Oberlin procedure versus MacKinnon technique (**Figure 2**) [8].

### 2.3 Intercostal nerves (ICN)

In 1968, Tsuyama and Hara suggested the transfer of two or more intercostal nerves (ICN) to the Musculo Cutaneous Nerve (MCN) [9]. In 1978, Celli neurotized torn roots of the brachial plexus (preliminary note on the surgical technique) [10]. In 1984, Dolenec performed various neurotizations using the ICN into MCN, radial, axilar or motor FG of ulnar nerve (sural nerve graft interposition) [11]. In 2003, Oberlin used an intercostal nerve transfer to neurotized triceps [12]. The transfer of ICN to MCN or to Radial nerve (long portion of triceps) are the 4-th choice. Each ICN presents approximately 1200 axons but we must not forget that: ICN 1 participates to the BP formation; ICN 2 is very small and with *no motor fibers*; ICN7 – ICN12 have very few motor axons - only up to 20%; ICN-3 to ICN-6 are used for neurotization of MCN;

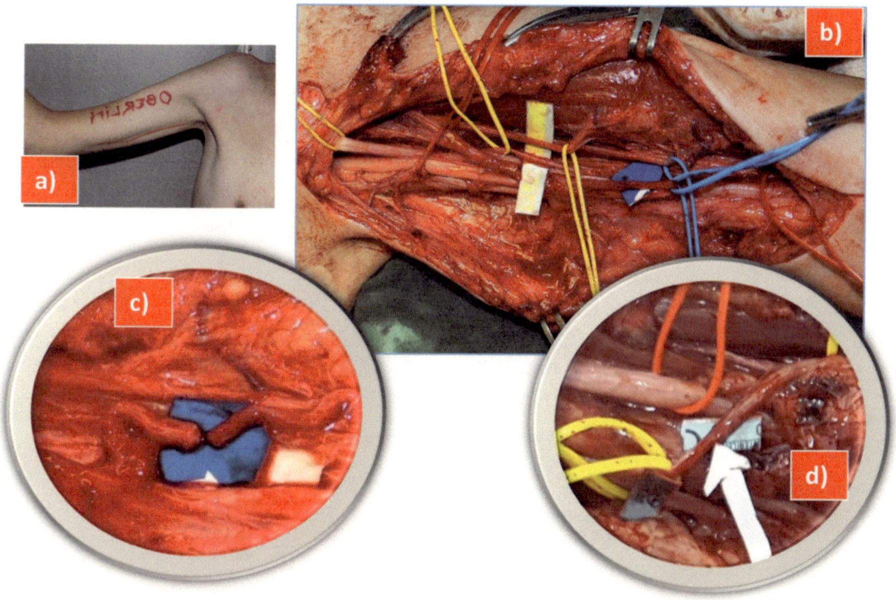


**Figure 1.**
*Oberlin technique: a) 8–10 cm incision, internal bicipital groove; b) MCN motor branch identification destined to the biceps, longitudinal epineurotomy 3–4 cm on the cubital nerve with the identification by electrostimulation of motor 2-FG; c) by internal neurolysis in the MCN trunk, the FG destined to the biceps are separated, sectioned at 3–4 cm proximally, the ends being transcended towards the ulnar nerve; the same procedure is done for the ulnar nerve FG, which are sectioned at 3–4 cm distally, so that the proximal transcended ends come in contact with the MCN FG ends; neuroraphy, motor FG from the UN to the MCN FG destined to the biceps, done without tension, with 3–4 points, nylon 9.0 or 10.0.*

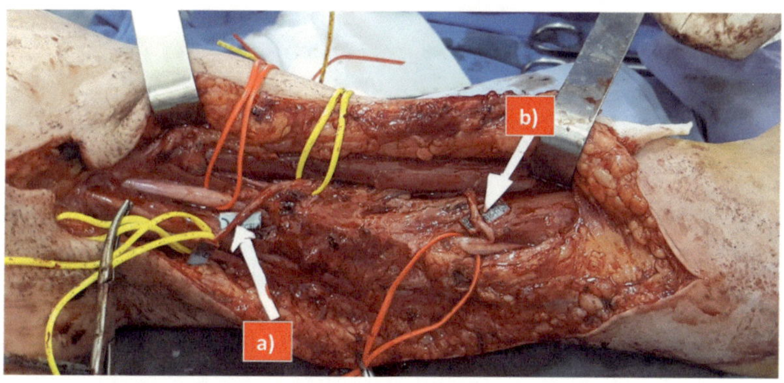


**Figure 2.**
*Mackinnon technique: a) Oberlin technique; b) FG isolated from the median nerve is connected to the MCN motor branch destined to the anterior brachial muscle [6].*

30–45% motor axons lose 10% of motor fibers to every 10 cm from the axillary line [4]. We prefer the surgical approach to harvest the ICN proposed by Hanno Millesi also used by David Chuang (**Figure 3**) [13]. ICN harvest is a technique requiring meticulous approach and careful dissection with proper hemostasis, preserving the serratus anterior muscle insertion [14]. We prefer the Oberlin technique because IC vasculo-nervous bundle is harvested without dissecting it, avoiding excessive bleeding (**Figure 4**) [15]. Minimal invasive robotic surgery has become possible today in centers equipped with surgical robot system - Da Vinci [16]. The ICN are connected to MCN by sural nerve graft (**Figure 5**). The indication of the NT with ICN are: 1) restoration of

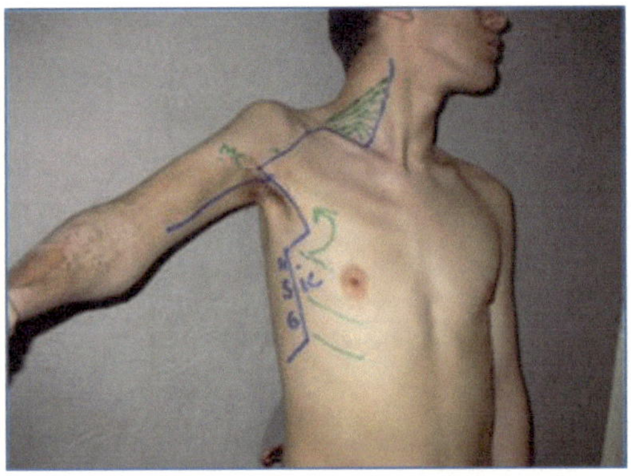

**Figure 3.**
*Intercostal nerves: Meticulous preoperative planning for the surgical approach.*

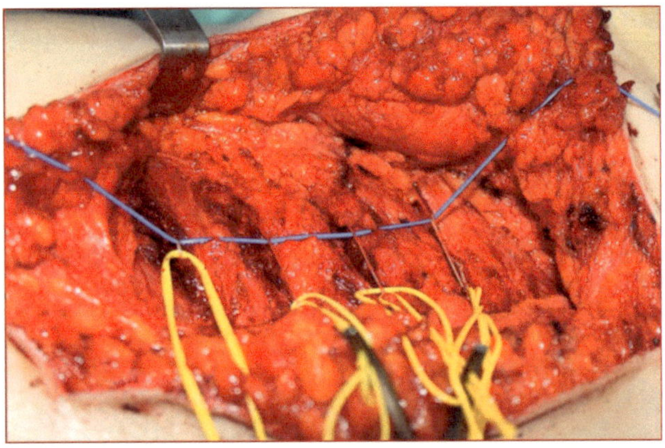

**Figure 4.**
*The intercostal nerves – Harvesting ICN technique: The dissection is difficult and with important bleeding; the Oberlin technique allows for the ICN isolation without major bleeding.*

elbow flexion is the first goal in brachial plexus injuries [17]; 2) ICN to the long head of the triceps nerve - for the restoration of elbow extension without nerve graft and afterwards, the reinnervated triceps can be transferred to the biceps (Carroll Technique); 3) gracilis free muscle transfer reinnerverted with ICN for elbow flexion [18]. We prefer to associate ICN transfer to MCN with Direct Neuro Muscular Neurotization (DNMN) to the denervated biceps and we consider that this improves the results (**Figure 6**).

The contraindications for ICN transfers are: ipsilateral phrenic nerve palsy, Serratus anterior muscle palsy or rib fractures [19]. The complications to use ICN are: 1) a variable degree of ipsilateral pulmonary atelectasis in infants [20]; 2) pleural rupture is in the opinion of some authors the most frequent complication [21].

## 2.4 Medial pectoral nerve (MPN)

MPN are 73% composed of fibers from C8 and T1, contains approximately 1,100 to 2,100 motor fibers, its surgically obtainable length is of up to 78 mm and has a mean diameter ranging between 1.4 and 2.7 mm [22]. The pectoral nerves - namely the lateral pectoral nerve (LPN) and the medial pectoral nerve (MPN) - are joined together by the pectoral loop. MPN innervates the lower pectoralis major and pectoralis minor muscle and may have connections to the intercostal

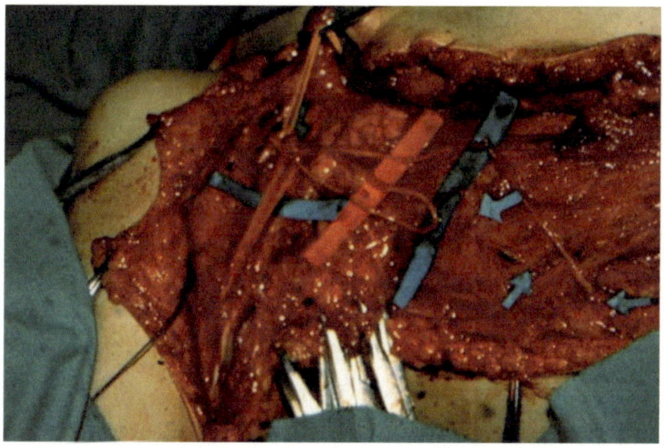

**Figure 5.**
*The intercostal nerves – connected to sural nerve graft: depending on the quality and length of the harvested sural nerve, 2 ICN may be connected or even one ICN to a sural nerve segment.*

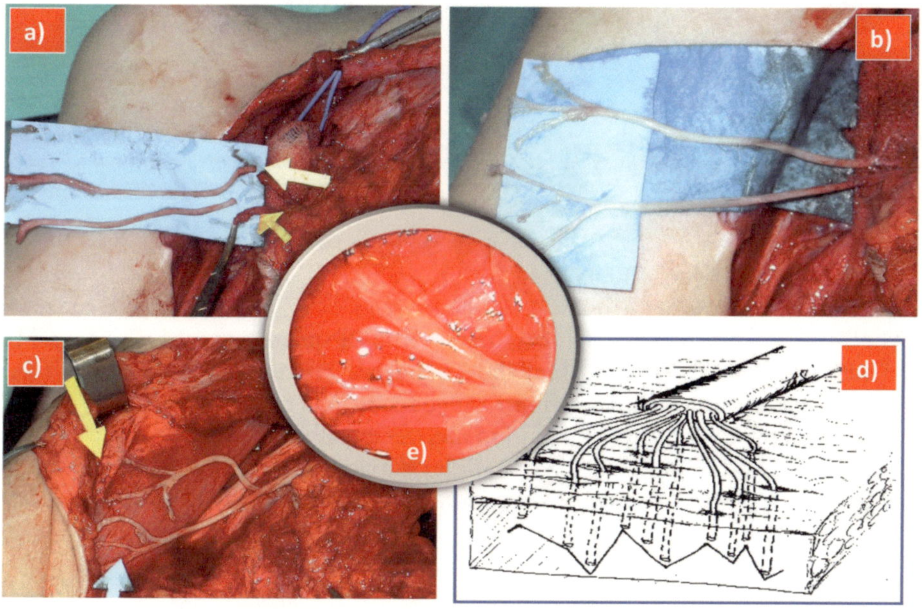


**Figure 6.**
*The intercostal nerves – direct neuro muscular neurotisation – giorgio Brunelli technique: (a) each ICN is connected to a sural nerve graft; b) the biceps extremity of each graft is opened wide c) the grafts must be long enough to allow arm abduction; d) the nerve fibers from each graft are inserted at different depths in the biceps muscle; e) a nylon 10.0 point is placed at the level between the perimysium and the epinerv to ensure stability.*

nerves [23]. The redundant innervation of the pectoralis major by the medial and lateral pectoral nerves allows for a continued pectoralis function after MPN transfer [7]. The MPN harvesting technique is relatively simple by a deltopectoral incision that highlights the infraclavicular plexus and the medial pectoral nerve is identified by electrostimulation; the branches of the medial pectoral nerve are sutured to the distal end of the branch from the biceps directly, without the interposition of a nerve graft. The MPN is dissected to obtain a sufficient length and is then sectioned; the MCN branch destined to the biceps is isolated on a sufficient length to allow a no tension neuroraphy with the MPN [24]. This transfer is indicated in patients with C 5,6 or C 5,6,7 lesions but with a good strength in the pectoralis major (**Figure 7**).

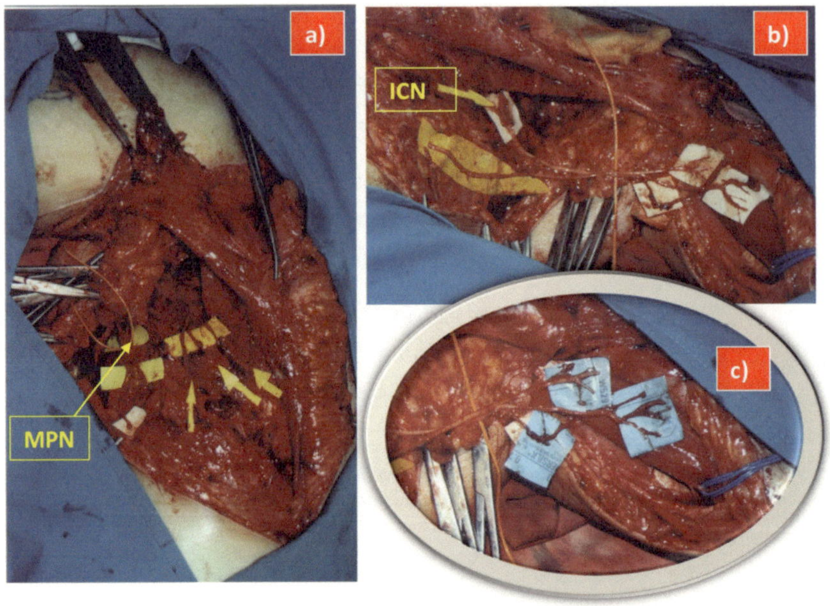


**Figure 7.**
*Medial pectoral nerve (MPN) to musculocutaneous nerve: a) MPN dissection and isolation to 2 ICN; b) connecting the sural nerve grafts between the MPN and the biceps branch from the MCN and each ICN with a graft which has been widened at the biceps extremity also for the DNMN Brunelli technique; c) double neurotization: MPN to MCN + ICN to biceps (DNMN).*

## 2.5 Thoracodorsal nerve (TDN)

The TDN is a motor nerve that originates from the posterior cord C7, C8 and less frequently C6-C8 [25]. The length of the TDN is 12.3 cm, the diameter ranges from 2.1 to 3.0 mm and the myelinated fibers range from 1530 to 2470.

TDN is a motor donor nerve useful in recovering elbow flexion without nerve grafting [26]. The TDN harvesting technique is made through an incision oriented at the level of the lateral border of the latissimus dorsi muscle with the upper limb

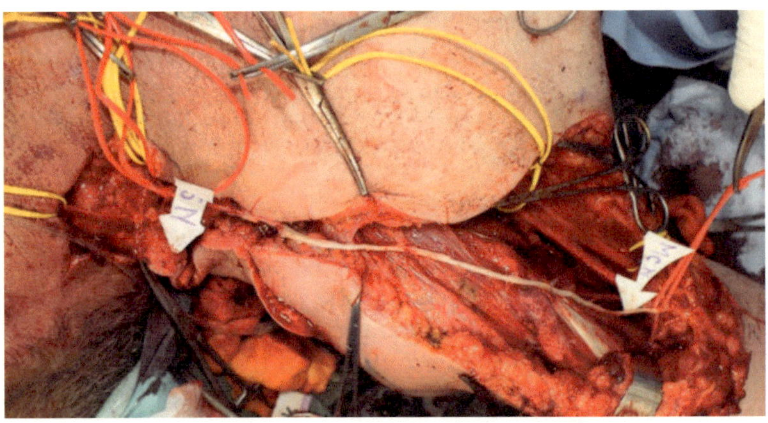

**Figure 8.**
*Spinal accessory nerve (SAN) to MCN: Motor FG from the SAN identified through electrostimulation were connected to a sural nerve graft which allows the connection to the biceps branch from the MCN avoiding retroclavicular dissection through scar tissue.*

at 90° abduction. After a distal to proximal MCN intraneural dissection, the TDN is connected to the FG of the MCN for the biceps muscle and to the FG for the brachialis muscle. TDN transfer to the MCN provides recovery of elbow flexion in 90% of cases [27]. TDN can be useful for neurotization of other nerves: axillary, suprascapular, spinal or anterior serratus [28].

### 2.6 Spinal accessory nerve (SAN)

The SAN contains approximately 1500 motor axons (C1 to C6) and was first used for MCN neurotization in 1980 by Marcelo Rosa de Rezende [29]. The SAN is harvested by an anterior approach for transfer to the MCN connected with a nerve graft (**Figure 8**) [30]. The posterior approach is used for transfer to the supra-scapular nerve (SSN) or associated with the triceps branch transfer to the axillary nerve [31]. Evaluating elbow flexion after SAN to MCN transfers have established MRC = M3 or better in 65–83% of patients [7].

### 2.7 Phrenic nerve (PhN)

In 1990, Chinese surgeons performed the first phrenic nerve transfers to the MCN to recover elbow flexion [32]. To avoid dissection through retroclavicular scar tissue we prefer in the transfer of the phrenic nerve to MCN a long bypass nerve graft of maximum 10 cm (**Figure 9**). PhN contains 800 myelinated motor axons (C3, C4, C5) and is a good donor nerve but we should not forget its contribution in the respiratory function [33]. Phrenic nerve (PhN) transfer to the MCN is not recommended in patients with previous pulmonary diseases or for children under the age of two years [29].

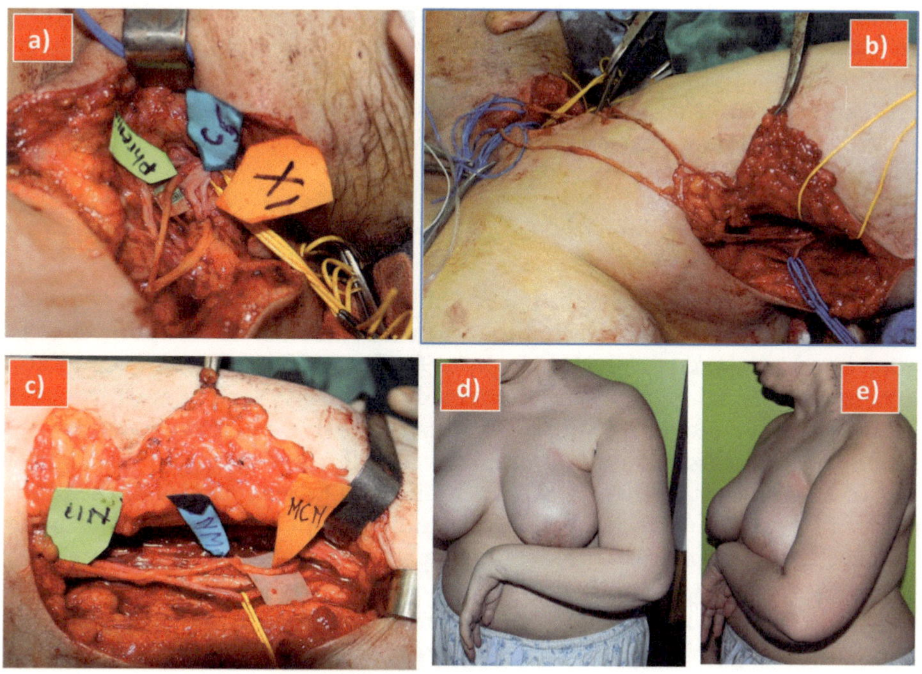


**Figure 9.**
*Phrenic nerve (**PhN**) to MCN: a) PhN, C5 root and ASN evidentiation; b) to avoid retroclavicular scar tissue area, we performed a long nerve grafts bypass; c) connecting the nerve grafts: PhN to MCN, C5 and ASN to MN and UN; d) and e) recovery of elbow flexion after 9 month.*

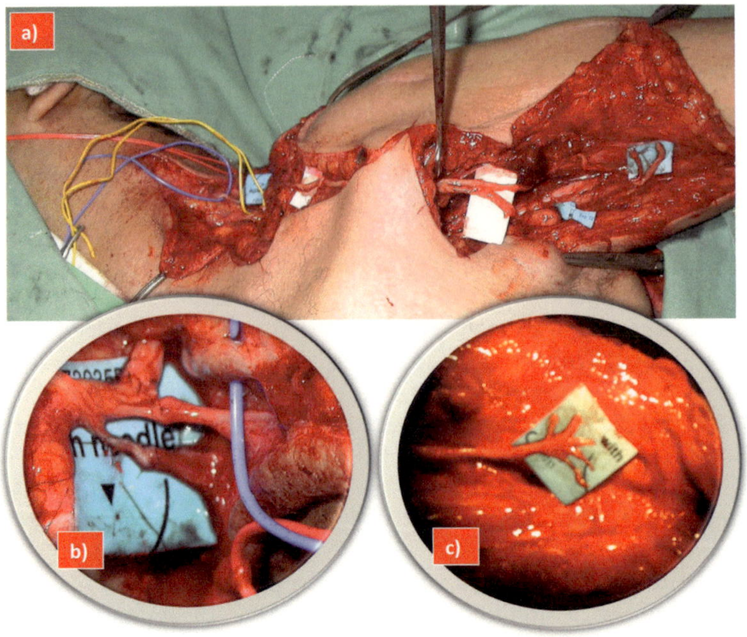


**Figure 10.**
*Cervical plexus + spinal accessory to MCN transfer; combined neurotisation (NNN + DNMN) by nerve graft C3 + C4 + SAN to MCN + biceps - a) dissection of the C3 and C4 anterior rami of the cervical plexus; b) proximal neurorraphy; c) DNMN associated.*

## 2.8 Cervical plexus C3-C4 to MCN

In 1984, Georgio Brunelli and Monini L. proposed to use the anterior motor branches of the cervical plexus. The anterior branches of the cervical plexus have approximately 14 000 myelinated axons but the distance of coaptation of the C3 and C4 anterior branches to the target (MCN) requires an intervening nerve graft [34]. We prefer to associate the transfer of anterior branches of cervical plexus with SAN and DNMN to MCN (**Figure 10**).

## 2.9 Contralateral C7 (CoC7) transfer to MCN

In 1992, a group of Chinese authors published the use of CoC7 and obtained good functional results considering that the procedure opens new perspectives in total brachial plexus paralysis [35]. In 1993, David Chuang used CoC7 as a source of neurotization, which he connected to the PB via a long graft from the sural nerve. After one year, in the second operative time, axonal growth was verified in the sural graft and neurorraphy was performed at MCN [36]. There are three different ways to harvest CoC7, including the whole root, 3/4 of the root and half (1/2) of the C7 root, respectively, and the functional recovery is much better in the whole root CoC7 transfer group - which provides a large number of donor nerve fibers - than that for the group with partial transfer [37]. CoC7 nerve transfer via a modified prespinal route and direct coaptation is not suitable because of the high complication rate: severe bleeding due to vertebral arterial injury during the procedure, temporary recurrent laryngeal nerve palsy, pain and numbness in the donor site during swallowing and dyspnea [38]. Because of the donor site morbidity after the (CoC7) transfer was relatively high, of over 20%, although the C7 has a large number of fibers (8467 ± 1019), it remains the last option [39].

## 3. Conclusions

Nerve transfer in elbow flexion recovery provides results. The choice of techniques in nervous surgery depends on: the type of lesion, the presence of the roots that can be grafted, the time between the accident and the intervention [4]. The association of the 3 methods: 1) neuro-neuronal neurotisation (NNN) = NT with 2) direct neuro-muscular neurotisation (DNMN) proposed by Georgio Brunelli to insert the nerve fibers at different levels in the muscle [40] and 3) teno-muscular transfer (TMT) improved the results in BPP [41].

## Conflict of interest

The authors declare no conflict of interest.

## Author details

Teodor Stamate and Dan Cristian Moraru*
University of Medicine and Pharmacy "Grigore T. Popa", Iași, Romania

*Address all correspondence to: morarudc@gmail.com

## References

[1] Narakas A. The surgical management of brachial plexus injuries. In: Daniel RK, Terzis JK, eds. Reconstructive microsurgery. Boston: Little, Brown and Co., 1977:443-460.

[2] Oberlin C, Béal D, Leechavengvongs S, Salon A, Dauge MC, Sarcy JJ. Nerve transfer to biceps muscle using a part of ulnar nerve for C5-C6 avulsion of the brachial plexus: anatomical study and report of four cases. J Hand Surg. 1994 Mar;19(2):232-237. doi: 10.1016/0363-5023(94)90011-6.

[3] Leechavengvongs S, Witoonchart K, Uerpairojkit C, Thuvasethakul P, Ketmalasiri W. Nerve transfer to biceps muscle using a part of the ulnar nerve in brachial plexus injury (upper arm type): a report of 32 cases. J Hand Surg Am. 1998 Jul;23(4):711-716. doi: 10.1016/S0363-5023(98)80059-2. PMID: 9708387.

[4] Teboul F, Goubier JN. Le plexus brachial et ses traumatismes. Création du site - 23/05/2008. https://www.plexusbrachial.com/qu-est-ce-qu-une-paralysie-du-plexus-brachial/

[5] Gutowski KA, Orenstein HH. Restoration of elbow flexion after brachial plexus injury: the role of nerve and muscle transfers. Plast Reconstr Surg. 2000 Nov;106(6):1348-1357; quiz 1358; discussion 1359. doi: 10.1097/00006534-200011000-00020. PMID: 11083569.

[6] Mackinnon SE, Novak CB, Myckatyn TM, Tung TH. Results of reinnervation of the biceps and brachialis muscles with a double fascicular transfer for elbow flexion. J Hand Surg Am. 2005 Sep;30(5):978-985. doi: 10.1016/j.jhsa.2005.05.014. PMID: 16182054.

[7] Ray WZ, Chang J, Hawasli A, Wilson TJ, Yang L. Motor Nerve Transfers: A Comprehensive Review. Neurosurgery. 2016 Jan;78(1):1-26. doi: 10.1227/NEU.0000000000001029. PMID: 26397751.

[8] Martins RS, Siqueira MG, Heise CO, Foroni L, Teixeira MJ. A prospective study comparing single and double fascicular transfer to restore elbow flexion after brachial plexus injury. Neurosurgery. 2013 May;72(5):709-714; discussion 714-5; quiz 715. doi: 10.1227/NEU.0b013e318285c3f6. PMID: 23313985.

[9] Tsuyama N, Hara T. Reconstructive surgery for traumatic braquial plexus injuries. Clin Orthop Surg. 1968; 3:675-687.

[10] Celli L, Balli A, de Luise G, Rovesta C. La neurotizzazione degli ultimi nervi intercostali, mediante trapianto nervoso peduncolato, nelle avulsioni radicolari del plesso brachiale. (Nota preliminare di tecnica chirurgica) [Neurotization of the last intercostal nerves, by peduncolated nerve graft, in torn roots of the brachial plexus (preliminary note on the surgical technic)]. Chir Organi Mov. 1978 Sep-Oct;64(5):461-4. Italian. PMID: 754906.

[11] Dolenc VV. Intercostal neurotization of the peripheral nerves in avulsion plexus injuries. Clin Plast Surg. 1984 Jan;11(1):143-147. PMID: 6705462.

[12] Oberlin C. Les paralysies du plexus brachial de l'adulte par lésions radiculaires, conception générale, orientations thérapeutiques et résultats [Brachial plexus palsy in adults with radicular lesions, general concepts, diagnostic approach and results ]. Chir Main. 2003 Dec;22(6):273-84. French. doi: 10.1016/j.main.2003.09.008. PMID: 14714505.

[13] Chuang DC, Yeh MC, Wei FC. Intercostal nerve transfer of the musculocutaneous nerve in avulsed brachial plexus injuries: evaluation of 66 patients. J Hand Surg Am. 1992

Sep;17(5):822-828. doi: 10.1016/0363-5023(92)90451-t. PMID: 1401789.

[14] Wahegaonkar AL, Doi K, Hattori Y, Addosooki AI. Technique of intercostal nerve harvest and transfer for various neurotization procedures in brachial plexus injuries. Tech Hand Up Extrem Surg. 2007 Sep;11(3):184-194. doi: 10.1097/bth.0b013e31804d44d2. PMID: 17805155.

[15] Oberlin C, Durand S, Belheyar Z, Shafi M, David E, Asfazadourian H. Nerve transfers in brachial plexus palsies. Chir Main. 2009 Feb;28 (1):1-9. doi: 10.1016/j.main.2008.11.010. PMID: 19162520.

[16] Liverneaux P, Berner SH, Bednar MS, et al. Telemicrosurgery: Robotic Assisted Microsurgery. 2013. Paris, France: Springer Verlag.

[17] Goubier JN, Teboul F, Khalifa H. Reanimation of elbow extension with intercostal nerves transfers in total brachial plexus palsies. Microsurgery. 2011 Jan;31(1):7-11. doi: 10.1002/micr.20822. Epub 2010 Nov 28. PMID: 21207492.

[18] Doi K. Management of total paralysis of the brachial plexus by the double free-muscle transfer technique. J Hand Surg Eur Vol. 2008 Jun;33(3):240-251. doi: 10.1177/1753193408090140. PMID: 18562352.

[19] Kovachevich R, Kircher MF, Wood CM, Spinner RJ, Bishop AT, Shin AY. Complications of intercostal nerve transfer for brachial plexus reconstruction. J Hand Surg Am. 2010 Dec;35(12):1995-2000. doi: 10.1016/j.jhsa.2010.09.013. Epub 2010 Nov 20. PMID: 21095076.

[20] El-Gammal TA, Abdel-Latif MM, Kotb MM, El-Sayed A, Ragheb YF, Saleh WR, Geith MA, Abdel-Ghaffar HS. Intercostal nerve transfer in infants with obstetric brachial plexus palsy. Microsurgery. 2008;28(7):499-504. doi: 10.1002/micr.20545. PMID: 18767133.

[21] de Mendonça Cardoso M, Gepp R, Lima FL, Gushiken A. Intercostal to musculocutaneous nerve transfer in patients with complete traumatic brachial plexus injuries: case series. Acta Neurochir (Wien). 2020 Aug;162(8):1907-1912. doi: 10.1007/s00701-020-04433-3. Epub 2020 Jun 6. PMID: 32506331.

[22] Lee KS. Anatomic variation of the spinal origins of lateral and medial pectoral nerves. Clin Anat. 2007 Nov;20(8):915-918. doi: 10.1002/ca.20556. PMID: 17948291.

[23] Porzionato A, Macchi V, Stecco C, Loukas M, Tubbs RS, De Caro R. Surgical anatomy of the pectoral nerves and the pectoral musculature. Clin Anat. 2012 Jul;25(5):559-575. doi: 10.1002/ca.21301. Epub 2011 Nov 28. PMID: 22125052.

[24] Brandt KE, Mackinnon SE. A technique for maximizing biceps recovery in brachial plexus reconstruction. J Hand Surg Am. 1993 Jul;18(4):726-733. doi: 10.1016/0363-5023(93)90328-Z. PMID: 8349991.

[25] Novak CB, Mackinnon SE, Tung TH. Patient outcome following a thoracodorsal to musculocutaneous nerve transfer for reconstruction of elbow flexion. Br J Plast Surg. 2002 Jul;55(5):416-419. doi: 10.1054/bjps.2002.3859. PMID: 12372371.

[26] Samardzic MM, Grujicic DM, Rasulic LG, Milicic BR. The use of thoracodorsal nerve transfer in restoration of irreparable C5 and C6 spinal nerve lesions. Br J Plast Surg. 2005 Jun;58(4):541-546. doi: 10.1016/j.bjps.2003.12.027. PMID: 15897040.

[27] Soldado F, Ghizoni MF, Bertelli J. Thoracodorsal nerve transfer for elbow flexion reconstruction in infraclavicular

brachial plexus injuries. J Hand Surg Am. 2014 Sep;39(9):1766-1770. doi: 10.1016/j.jhsa.2014.04.043. Epub 2014 Jun 13. PMID: 24934602.

[28] Potter SM, Ferris SI. Vascularized Thoracodorsal to Suprascapular Nerve Transfer, a Novel Technique to Restore Shoulder Function in Partial Brachial Plexopathy. Front Surg. 2016 Mar 14;3:17. doi: 10.3389/fsurg.2016.00017. PMID: 27014699; PMCID: PMC4789804.

[29] Rezende MR, Silva GB, Paula EJ, Mattar Junior R, Camargo OP. What has changed in brachial plexus surgery? Clinics (Sao Paulo). 2013;68(3):411-8. doi: 10.6061/clinics/2013(03)r02. PMID: 23644864; PMCID: PMC3611894.

[30] Bertelli JA, Ghizoni MF. Results of spinal accessory to suprascapular nerve transfer in 110 patients with complete palsy of the brachial plexus. J Neurosurg Spine. 2016 Jun;24(6):990-995. doi: 10.3171/2015.8.SPINE15434. Epub 2016 Feb 12. PMID: 26871649.

[31] Bhandari PS, Deb P. Posterior approach for both spinal accessory nerve to suprascapular nerve and triceps branch to axillary nerve for upper plexus injuries. J Hand Surg Am. 2013 Jan;38(1):168-172. doi: 10.1016/j.jhsa.2012.10.024. PMID: 23261196.

[32] Gu YD, Wu MM, Zhen YL, Zhao JA, Zhang GM, Chen DS, Yan JQ, Cheng XM. Phrenic nerve transfer for treatment of root avulsion of the brachial plexus. Chin Med J (Engl). 1990 Apr;103(4):267-270. PMID: 2118036.

[33] Sakellariou VI, Badilas NK, Stavropoulos NA, Mazis G, Kotoulas HK, Kyriakopoulos S, Tagkalegkas I, Sofianos IP. Treatment options for brachial plexus injuries. ISRN Orthop. 2014 Apr 14;2014:314137. doi: 10.1155/2014/314137. PMID: 24967125; PMCID: PMC4045367.

[34] Brunelli G, Monini L. Neurotization of avulsed roots of brachial plexus by means of anterior nerves of cervical plexus. Clinics in Plastic Surgery. 1984 Jan;11(1):149-152. DOI:10.1201/9780429265822-24

[35] Gu YD, Zhang GM, Chen DS, Yan JG, Cheng XM, Chen L. Seventh cervical nerve root transfer from the contralateral healthy side for treatment of brachial plexus root avulsion. J Hand Surg Br. 1992 Oct;17(5):518-521. doi: 10.1016/s0266-7681(05)80235-9. PMID: 1479244.

[36] Chuang DC, Wei FC, Noordhoff MS. Cross-chest C7 nerve grafting followed by free muscle transplantations for the treatment of total avulsed brachial plexus injuries: a preliminary report. Plast Reconstr Surg. 1993 Sep;92(4):717-725; discussion 726-7. PMID: 8356134.

[37] Gao Km, Hu Jj, Lao J, Zhao X. Evaluation of nerve transfer options for treating total brachial plexus avulsion injury: A retrospective study of 73 participants. Neural Regen Res 2018;13: 470-476, DOI: 10.4103/1673-5374.228730

[38] Li W, Wang S, Zhao J, Rahman MF, Li Y, Li P, Xue Y. Complications of contralateral C-7 transfer through the modified prespinal route for repairing brachial plexus root avulsion injury: a retrospective study of 425 patients. J Neurosurg. 2015 Jun;122(6):1421-1428. doi: 10.3171/2014.10.JNS131574. Epub 2014 Dec 12. PMID: 25495742.

[39] Yang G, Chang KW, Chung KC. A Systematic Review of Contralateral C7 Transfer for the Treatment of Traumatic Brachial Plexus Injury: Part 1. Overall Outcomes. Plast Reconstr Surg. 2015 Oct;136(4):794-809. doi: 10.1097/PRS.0000000000001494. PMID: 26397253; PMCID: PMC4602165.

[40] Brunelli G. Direct neurotization of severely damaged muscles. J Hand Surg Am. 1982;7:572-579. [PubMed] [Google Scholar]

[41] Stamate T, Budurca AR, Lazar AN, Tamas C, Stamate M. Results in brachial plexus palsy after biceps neuro-muscular neurotization associated with neuro-neural neurotization and teno-muscular transfer. Acta Neurochir Suppl. 2005;93:141-145. doi: 10.1007/3-211-27577-0_24. PMID: 15986744.

Chapter 3

# Nerve Transfers to Recover External Rotation of the Shoulder after Brachial Plexus Injuries in Adults

*Jean-Noel Goubier, Camille Echalier, Elodie Dubois and Frédéric Teboul*

## Abstract

Restoration of external rotation of the shoulder in adults with partial brachial plexus palsies is challenging. While nerve grafts are possible, nerve transfers are currently the most use method for satisfactory restoration of function. Numerous nerve transfers have been described, although the transfer of the spinal accessory nerve to the suprascapular nerve remains the gold standard. The suprascapular nerve and the nerve to the teres minor muscle are the two preferred targets to restore external rotation of the shoulder. There are numerous nerve donors, but their use obviously depends on the initial injury. The most common donors are the spinal accessory nerve, the rhomboid nerve, branches of the radial nerve, the C7 root fascicle or the ulnar nerve. The choice for the transfer depends on the available nerves and first of all on chosen approach, whether it be cervical or scapular. It also depends on the other associated reconstruction procedures, grafts, or nerve transfers for the recovery of other functions, specifically, elevation of the shoulder and flexion of the elbow. The objective of this chapter is to present the main nerve transfers and to propose a therapeutic strategy.

**Keywords:** Brachial plexus injury, nerve transfers, shoulder external rotation

## 1. Introduction

Restoration of external rotation of the shoulder in brachial plexus palsies is challenging. This function, however, is necessary for properly orienting the upper limb for the movements needed in everyday life. While flexion of the elbow and elevation of the shoulder are prioritized for restoration, external rotation of the shoulder should not be neglected. Most of the time, it can be achieved at the same time of operation if nerve transfers are used.

The two nerves mainly targeted for the recovery of this function are the suprascapular nerve (SSN) innervating the infraspinatus external rotator muscle and the branch of the axillary nerve innervating the teres minor external rotator muscle. Several nerve transfers could be proposed due to the large number and variety of lesions of the brachial plexus roots.



IntechOpen

## 2. Most used nerve transfers

### 2.1 Transfer of the spinal accessory nerve to the suprascapular nerve

Transfer of the spinal accessory nerve (SAN) to the suprascapular nerve (SSN) remains the gold standard for restoring external rotation to the shoulder with nerve transfer (**Figure 1**). This transfer can be carried out in all partial or complete palsies of the brachial plexus, as long as the spinal nerve has not been damaged, which is the case for 96% of brachial plexus injuries [1]. A testing of the trapezius muscle strength is needed before carrying out this transfer. If the trapezius is not scored at least M4, this transfer cannot be undertaken.

This transfer could be carried out via an anterior cervical approach [1] or a posterior scapular approach [2]. The anterior approach is essentially used in the case of a complete palsy of the brachial plexus where an exploration and an possible associated root graft is envisaged. A classical transversal approach of exploration of the plexus may be used as well as the extended approach described by Bertelli [1], allowing improved results with respect to external rotation and abduction of the shoulder. When the anterior cervical approach is used, the anterior branch of the spinal nerve is released and sutured to the origin of the SSN at the beginning of the primary trunk. If the root injury is more distal, the primary trunk may be damaged, and the dissection of the SSN may be difficult, if not impossible. In that case, the suture needs to be made more distally at the level of the coracoid notch and the extended approach of Bertelli [3] becomes necessary.

The results for external rotation were 87 degrees of rotation from the thorax in 40% of patients in a series of 81 patients (**Table 1**). It seems that even with a perfectly optimized nerve transfer, the results are only satisfactory for half of the series.

Certain authors have described, in a case report, the use of the contralateral SAN for SSN restoration using an intercalated graft [4]. The results after 12 months were weak (3 degrees of external rotation), presumably because the use of a graft reduces

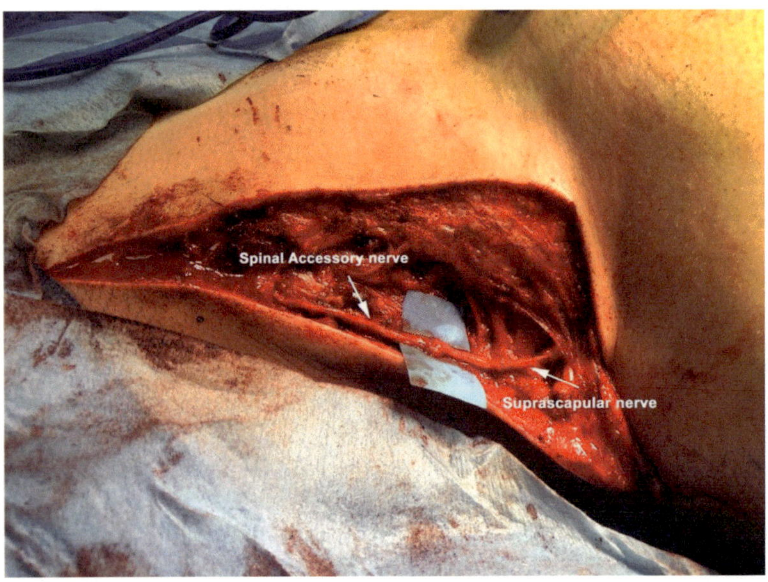


**Figure 1.**
*Transfer of the spinal accessory nerve to the suprascapular nerve in the cervical region by an anterior approach. This approach allows restoration of external rotation and treatment of other deficient functions using grafts of non-avulsed roots (right side).*

| Donor nerve | Targeted nerve | Author, year | N | Follow up (months) | External Rotation | Time to surgery (months) |
|---|---|---|---|---|---|---|
| Spinal accessory | Suprascapular nerve | Bertelli, 2016 [1] | 81 | 40 (SD 14) | 0° - 60% | 5,2 (SD 2,4) |
| | | | | | 87° (SD 40,6°) - 40% | |
| | | Zermeno-Rivera, 2015 [4] | Case report | 12 | 3° | — |
| | | Yin, 2012 [5] | 3 | 39,2 | 60° - 70° | 4,6 (SD 3,3) |
| Branch for the rhomboid muscle | | Goubier, 2020 [6] | 8 | 32 (25 to 48) | 70° to 80° - 38% | — |
| | | | | | 90° - 38% | |
| | | | | | 100° to 110° - 25% | |
| Branch of the Radial nerve for the triceps | Nerve for the infraspinatus muscle | Tavares, [7] | 9 | 36 | 0° - 23% | 6,5 |
| | | | | | 20° to 45° - 44% | |
| | | | | | 90° - 11% | |
| | | | | | 120° - 11% | |
| | | | | | 1 lost of follow up | |
| Fascicule of the C7 root | Suprascapular nerve | Bertelli, 2004 [8] (Contralateral C7 root) | 12 (partial palsy) | 36 | 92° (range 80°-120°) | 4,3 (range 2–6) |
| | | | 12 (total palsy) | | 75° (range 40° - 100°) - 17% | |
| | | | | | 0° - 83% | |
| | | Yin, 2012 [5] (Fascicules of ipsilateral C7 root combined with transfer to post div of the upper trunk) | 5 | 39,2 | 0° | 4,6 (SD 3,3) |

**Table 1.**
*Summary of clinical results (external shoulder rotation) stratified by nerve transfer.*

the possibility of a direct nerve transfer by reducing the results in terms of delay and extent of recovery. In addition, the exploration and sacrifice of a nerve from the healthy side may be discussed for a brachial plexus palsy.

### 2.2 Transfer of the rhomboid nerve to the suprascapular nerve

This technique may be used for partial and complete injuries of the brachial plexus [6, 9, 10]. The rhomboid nerve branches comes from the dorsal scapular nerve, the posterior branch of C5. This branch starts relatively proximally and can be damaged in the case of an avulsion of C5. However, it receives the afferents from the C4 root and could, in theory, be used even in the case of an avulsion of the C5 root. The main indication for the rhomboid nerve transfer is a lesion of the SAN. In this case, the transfer could be associated with a transfer of the teres minor nerve from the long triceps nerve or a fascicle of the ulnar nerve (**Figures 2** and **3**).

The rhomboid nerve can be sutured directly to the SSN in the supraspinatus fossa. This technique is carried out using the posterior approach; the suture is close to the infraspinatus muscle, thus encouraging a more rapid recovery. In addition, the posterior dissection eliminates a lesion of the SSN in its passage under the notch and limits the risk of failure of a more proximal suture. The results from our series show that external rotation is recovered. The extent of the results, however, is a little bit less than that of a transfer from the spinal nerve (**Table 1**) [6].

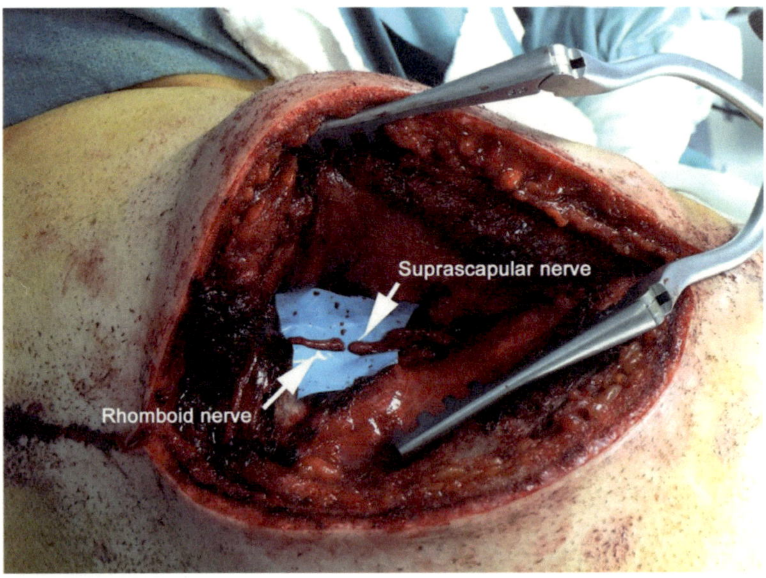


**Figure 2.**
*Transfer of the rhomboid nerve to the suprascapular nerve: The levator scapulae is released from the medial border of the scapula to expose the dorsal scapular nerve. The nerve to the rhomboid muscle is released until it reaches the upper edge of the rhomboid muscle, divided, and then turned toward the suprascapular nerve in the supraspinatus fossa (right shoulder) (courtesy of Elsevier [9]).*

### 2.3 Transfer of the long head of the triceps nerve to the teres minor nerve

This nerve transfer only applies to cases where there are partial lesions of the brachial plexus with preservation of a triceps scored at least M4. This technique is best suited to an axillary approach. The branch of the radial nerve leading to the

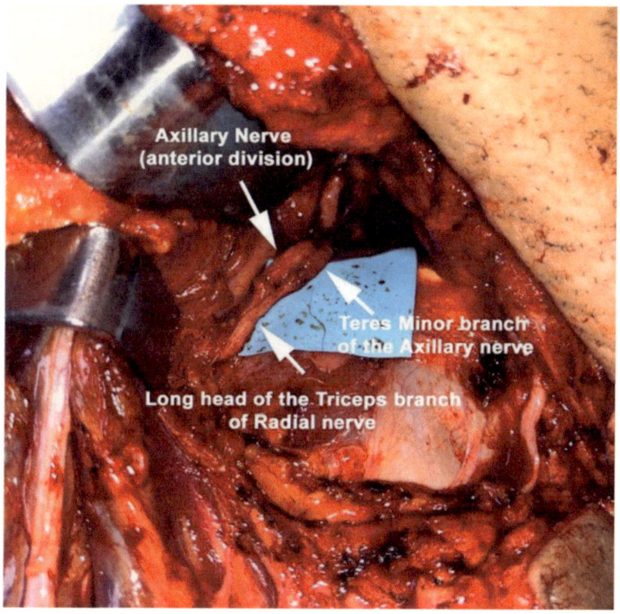


**Figure 3.**
*Transfer of the rhomboid nerve to the suprascapular nerve with a posterior approach (right shoulder). This transfer can be performed without any tension. With this approach, the nerve is sutured close to the supraspinatus muscle, encouraging faster recovery (courtesy of Elsevier [10]).*

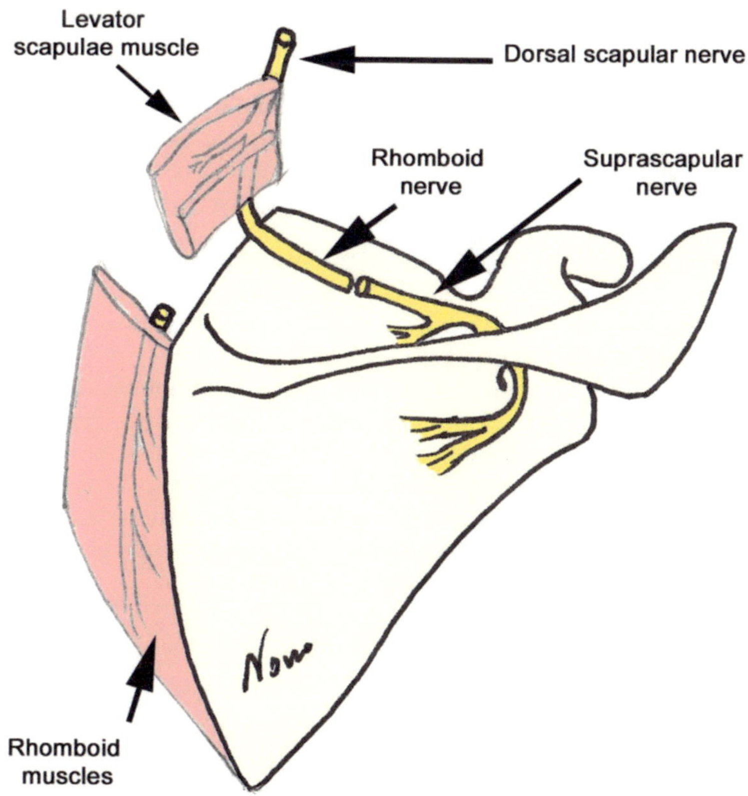


**Figure 4.**
*Transfer of the radial nerve (long head of the triceps branch) to the anterior division of the axillary nerve and to teres minor branch by an axillary approach (right axilla).*

triceps is easily identified because it is the first branch; electrostimulation clearly confirms with contraction of the long head of the triceps muscle. The axillary nerve is identified in the axillary fossa and the branch for the teres minor is isolated and separated from the axillary nerve. This branch is divided as distally as possible, then turned back toward the nerve of the long head of the triceps. The suture is generally made without tension (**Figure 4**).

The results for external rotation seem less satisfactory with this transfer than for the transfer of the spinal nerve. The teres minor is more of an accessory muscle for external rotation than the infraspinatus muscle [11]. The axon count showed that the number of fascicles in the branches of the radial nerve is less than the sum of fascicles in the axillary nerve and teres minor nerve. For this reason, some authors propose to use several branches of the radial nerve to optimize the number of fascicles transferred to the trunk of the axillary nerve and its branches (in particular the nerve of the teres minor) [12].

## 3. Other less used transfers

### 3.1 Transfer of a branch of the radial nerve to the infraspinatus muscle

This described transfer is anatomically possible. However, it does not seem to give satisfactory results for external rotation according to the authors [7] (**Table 1**). As a result, the authors do not recommend this transfer.

### 3.2 Transfer of a fascicle of the ulnar nerve to the teres minor nerve

This nerve transfer also only applies to cases where there are partial lesions of the brachial plexus and where a hand without palsy confirms the integrity of the ulnar nerve. One or two fascicles may have already been used to restore flexion of the elbow. Using additional ulnar fascicles could lead to a subsequent palsy with loss of grasp strength which would be very negative for the patient. The indication of this transfer should be considered with caution in the case of shoulder and elbow palsy.

### 3.3 Transfer of a fascicle of the C7 root to the suprascapular nerve

This transfer was proposed by Bertelli in 2004 using the contralateral C7 root [8] and by Yin et al. in 2012 using the ipsilateral C7 root [5]. The latter proposed to use a fascicle of C7 in order to restore the suprascapular nerve when the spinal nerve was not functional [5] (**Table 1**). The advantage of the ipsilateral transfer is that it can be carried out directly in the supraclavicular fossa and therefore is fully adapted if other procedures are carried out, especially a graft from the C5 or C6 roots if they are not avulsed. It should be noted that the damage to the spinal nerve during violent and prolonged trauma to the brachial plexus is generally associated with root avulsions, thus limiting this technique.

## 4. How to choose a transfer?

Prior to concluding that nerve transfer is indicated, the glenohumeral joint must obviously be assessed in order to rule out osteoarticular pathology that could mechanically limit the external rotation of the shoulder (joint malunion, gleno-humeral osteoarthritis, foreign bodies, etc). For this, imaging is necessary, such as simple standard x-rays of the shoulder or by performing arthrography of the glenohumeral joint (**Figure 5**).

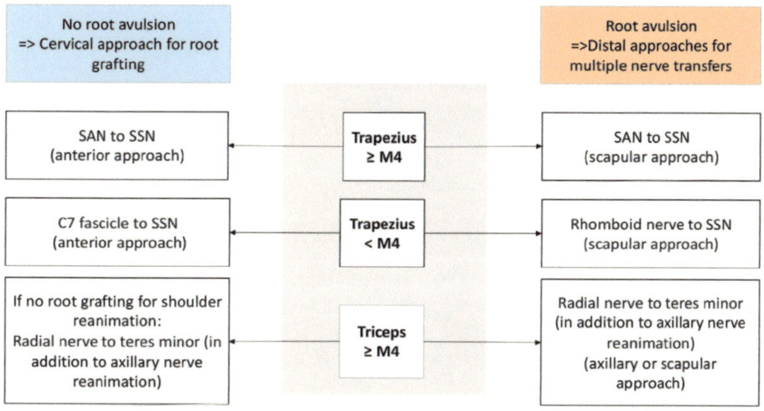


**Figure 5.**
*Decision tree to choose the best nerve transfer for restoration of external rotation in adults with brachial plexus palsies. Trapezius and triceps muscles must be tested to assess the function of the spinal accessory nerve and the radial nerve, respectively. (SAN: Spinal accessory nerve; SSN: Suprascapular nerve.)*

If a mechanical joint problem exists, it must be resolved before the nerve surgery if possible. In addition, glenohumeral arthrodesis can also be considered, allowing joint pathology and restoration of external rotation to be treated at the same time [13].

The choice of transfer depends primarily on the donor nerves available but also on the approaches used. If a cervical exploration of the plexus is chosen to carry out grafts (no root avulsions), in order to restore other functions, the use of the SAN (if the trapezius is functional) or of the fascicles from C7 root could be used with a direct suture on the SSN at its origin from the primary trunk, or by an extended approach at its entrance under the transverse coracoid ligament in order to improve results [1]. A distal transfer of a branch of the radial nerve (if the triceps is functional) to the teres minor could also be associated with this procedure in order to improve the results. If cervical exploration is not necessary (root avulsions), the use of the rhomboid nerve [9] (generally preserved even if the C5 root is avulsed), or of the SAN (if the trapezius is functional) by the posterior approach is preferred. In this context, a second distal transfer to the teres minor is rarely possible because if the C7 root is avulsed, the branches from the triceps are generally not functional, but in any case, the triceps must be tested because anatomical variations are possible.

## 5. Conclusion

The restoration of external rotation by nerve transfer is frequently possible because of numerous transfer possibilities. The use of one type of transfer or another depends on the reanimation strategy, on carrying out a cervical exploration and on other transfers used. A double transfer for external rotation can be generally also proposed.

The results, however, are often limited in terms of range-of-motion, even when the technique is carried out perfectly. Obviously, it is important to not forget the use of palliative muscle transfers, especially the transfer of the latissimus dorsi to the rotator cuff or the transfer of the lower part of the trapezius [14], if their innervation is preserved, or in the case of failure of the nerve surgery. Finally, for some, performing an arthrodesis on the shoulder will permit reestablishment of a superior external rotation compared with nerve transfers [13, 15].

## Conflict of interest

"The authors declare no conflict of interest."

## Author details

Jean-Noel Goubier[1*], Camille Echalier[2], Elodie Dubois[1] and Frédéric Teboul[1]

1 Nerve and Brachial Plexus Surgery Institute, Paris, France

2 Nollet Institute, Paris, France

*Address all correspondence to: jngoubier@gmail.com

## References

[1] Bertelli JA, Ghizoni MF. Results of spinal accessory to suprascapular nerve transfer in 110 patients with complete palsy of the brachial plexus. J Neurosurg Spine. 2016;24(6):990-995.

[2] Bhandari PS, Deb P. Dorsal approach in transfer of the distal spinal accessory nerve into the suprascapular nerve: histomorphometric analysis and clinical results in 14 cases of upper brachial plexus injuries. J Hand Surg Am. 2011;36(7):1182-1190.

[3] Bertelli JA, Ghizoni MF. Refinements in the technique for repair of the accessory nerve. J Hand Surg Am. 2006;31(8):1401-1406.

[4] Zermeno-Rivera J, Gutierrez-Amavizca BE. Contralateral Spinal Accessory Nerve Transfer: A New Technique in Panavulsive Brachial Plexus Palsy. Indian J Surg. 2015;77(3):247-250.

[5] Yin HW, Jiang S, Xu WD, Xu L, Xu JG, Gu YD. Partial ipsilateral C7 transfer to the upper trunk for C5-C6 avulsion of the brachial plexus. Neurosurgery. 2012;70(5):1176-1181; discussion 81-2.

[6] Goubier JN, Echalier C, Dubois E, Teboul F. Transfer of the rhomboid nerve for restoration of shoulder external rotation in partial brachial plexus palsy. Injury. 2020;51 Suppl 4:S84-SS7.

[7] Tavares PL, Siqueira MG, Martins RS, Zaccariotto M, Foroni L, Heise CO, et al. Restoration of shoulder external rotation by means of the infraspinatus muscle reinnervation with a radial nerve branch transfer. Br J Neurosurg. 2020;34(5):552-558.

[8] Bertelli JA, Ghizoni MF. Contralateral motor rootlets and ipsilateral nerve transfers in brachial plexus reconstruction. J Neurosurg. 2004;101(5):770-778.

[9] Goubier JN, Teboul F. Transfer of the rhomboid nerve to the suprascapular nerve: An anatomical feasibility study. Chir Main. 2015;34(4):182-185.

[10] Goubier JN, Teboul F. Rhomboid nerve transfer to the suprascapular nerve for shoulder reanimation in brachial plexus palsy: A clinical report. Hand Surg Rehabil. 2016;35(5):363-366.

[11] Elhassan B, Bishop A, Shin A, Spinner R. Shoulder tendon transfer options for adult patients with brachial plexus injury. J Hand Surg Am. 2010;35(7):1211-1219.

[12] Khair MM, Schreiber JJ, Rosenblatt L, Byun DJ, Lee SK, Wolfe SW. Axon Counts Yield Multiple Options for Triceps Fascicular Nerve to Axillary Nerve Transfer. J Hand Surg Am. 2016;41(11):e405-ee10.

[13] Degeorge B, Lazerges C, Chammas PE, Coulet B, Lacombe F, Chammas M. Comparison of spinal accessory nerve transfer to suprascapular nerve vs. shoulder arthrodesis in adults with brachial plexus injury. Orthop Traumatol Surg Res. 2019;105(8):1555-1561.

[14] Bertelli JA. Upper and lower trapezius muscle transfer to restore shoulder abduction and external rotation in longstanding upper type palsies of the brachial plexus in adults. Microsurgery. 2011;31(4):263-267.

[15] Chammas M, Goubier JN, Coulet B, Reckendorf GM, Picot MC, Allieu Y. Glenohumeral arthrodesis in upper and total brachial plexus palsy. A comparison of functional results. J Bone Joint Surg Br. 2004;86(5):692-695.

Chapter 4

# Derotational Osteotomies for The Late Treatment of Brachial Plexus Injury

*Ahmet Emrah Açan and Ertuğrul Şahin*

## Abstract

Obstetric brachial plexus palsy [OBBP] can affect the function of the upper extremity. Most of the injuries are limited to the upper spinal nerves and heals spontaneously. However, some of them will have incomplete recovery after OBBP often results in weakness of the external rotators [teres minor and infraspinatus] muscles compared to the internal rotators [teres major, pectoralis major, latissimus dorsi] muscles. The predominance of the internal rotators and adductor muscles over external rotators leads to an internal rotation contracture. The development of internal rotational deformity may progress to increased glenoid retroversion and posterior humeral head subluxation. If the surgeon does not repair internal rotation deformity, the humeral head is forced into a posterior position causing a complete posterior dislocation. Many procedures are performed to treat these deformities: In the young child, improving the remodeling of the glenohumeral joint, capsulectomy, and subscapular release are introduced. Tendon transfers of the shoulder have good results for motion but fail to restore the glenohumeral joint. The failure of improving joint alignment may represent the loss in clinical improvement over time. In older children, a humeral osteotomy can be an alternative to realign the limb into external rotation, improve appearance, and enhance eating, washing hair, and scratching the back of the neck. We will discuss all the techniques along with their advantages and disadvantages.

**Keywords:** brachial plexus, birth palsy, humeral rotation, glenohumeral join, osteotomy, technique

## 1. Introduction

Obstetric brachial plexus palsy (OBBP) can substantially impact the function of the upper extremity. The widely agreed-upon mechanism of the birth injury for brachial plexus is a combination of traction and lateral pressure on the head through the late stages of a difficult delivery. The shoulders can be stacked in the birth canal. Partial or complete ruptures of the nerves in the plexus area can occur during that traction.

Most of the injuries are limited to the upper spinal nerves, and the possibility of spontaneous healing is higher than the others [1–3]. The definition of 'Erb-Duchenne palsy' or 'Erb's palsy refers to a C5-C6 injury that results in the paralysis of the shoulder and elbow flexion. In addition, paralyzes of wrist and finger extensors can be accomplished, and it shows that C7 is also injured. Most of these partial plexus injuries have a good prognosis, and 70–80% recover spontaneously [4, 5].

However, incomplete recovery after brachial plexus birth palsy often results in weak external rotators [teres minor and infraspinatus] muscles compared to the internal rotators [teres major, pectoralis major, latissimus dorsi] muscles. The predominance of the internal rotators and adductor muscles over external rotators leads to an internal rotation contracture. The development of internal rotational deformity may progress to early glenohumeral joint deformity by six months of age and advanced deformity by two years, which is characterized by increased glenoid retroversion and posterior humeral head subluxation [6–10]. If this internal rotation deformity is not repaired, the humeral head is forced into a posterior position, causing an initial subluxation that can evolve to complete posterior dislocation. This condition was thought to be rare.

Many studies have shown that the onset of glenoid dysplasia with obstetric brachial plexus palsy occurs at an earlier age than previously recognized. The prevalence of this problem may have been underestimated [11–13]. Zancolli et al. [14] reported that this posterior dislocation occurs in 8% of patients with proximal humeral deformities and muscle contractures.

Several studies have reported glenoid and humeral pathology in cases of Erb's palsy [7, 8, 15, 16]. Waters et al. [8] defined the seven types for the glenohumeral deformity with OBBP (type I: normal articulation; type II: glenoid retroversion <5 degrees with no subluxation; type III: posterior subluxation; type IV: progressive posterior humeral subluxation into a pseudo-glenoid; type V: advance flattening of the humeral head and glenoid, with progressive or complete posterior dislocation of the humeral head; type VI: dislocation of the glenohumeral joint in infancy and type VII: growth arrest of the proximal part of the humerus). Pearl et al. [15] classified the glenoid deformity in patients with Erb's palsy as concentric, concentric-posterior, flat, bi-concave, and pseudoglenoid. Zancolli et al. [17] reported that a posterior epiphysiolysis of the proximal humerus caused the retroversion of the humeral head.

## 2. History

Surgical treatment of obstetric plexus lesions began with nerve repairs in 1902 [18] by Kennedy. However, long-term treatment results showed that partially healed birth injuries developed deformities, especially in the shoulders and elbows, and thus surgeons began to find an alternative surgical treatment. The aim of these procedures is to improve the function of a deformed extremity after a partially recovered nerve lesion. Release of tendons and muscles were defined to improve the function and range of motion in the early 20th century [2, 19]. Muscle transfers to improve the strength of the joints, not functional enough, were performed in the 1930s [20]. Surgeons preferred osteotomy techniques for improving the function and motion range of limbs. Thus surgeons hoped that patients could receive a functional level that would be able to cope with daily activities by themselves [21].

To this date, the treatment is controversial. Many procedures are performed to prevent or to treat these deformities: In the young child, improving the remodeling of the glenohumeral joint, capsulectomy, and subscapular release are introduced to reduce the pressure over the glenohumeral joint [22–24]. Tendon transfers of the shoulder have good results for motion but fail to restore the glenohumeral joint [25, 26]. The failure of improving joint alignment may represent the loss in clinical

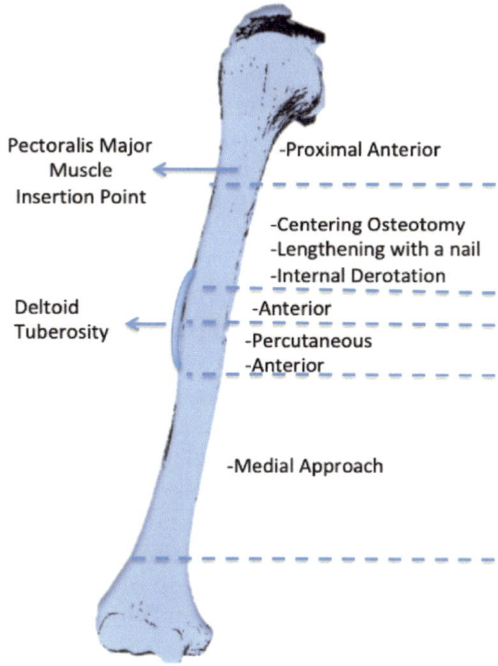


**Figure 1.**
*Demonstration of osteotomy techniques according to the location on the humerus. Dashed lines indicated the border of the defined osteotomy site.*

improvement over time [27]. In the older child, it is impossible to reduce the glenohumeral joint. In addition, traumatic brachial plexus injuries in adults can result in the shoulder joint's internal rotational deformity. Humeral osteotomy can be an alternative in both adults and children to realign the limb into external rotation, improve appearance, and enhance activities of daily living, such as eating, washing hair, and scratching the back of the neck [28–30]. Multiple techniques have been described for osteotomy of the humerus. Zancolli et al. [31] performed osteotomy with low axillar incision and at the just distal to the insertion point of the pectoralis major muscle. Glez Cuesta et al. [32] and Goddard et al. [33] performed the osteotomy just above the deltoid insertion via deltopectoral approach. Al Zahrani [34] performed the osteotomy just below the deltoid insertion. Briefly, different osteotomy levels have been described for each technique (**Figure 1**). We will discuss all the techniques along with their advantages and disadvantages in this chapter.

## 3. Patient evaluation

Preoperatively, the ability of the patients to perform activities of daily living (feeding, washing, and cleaning themselves) with the functionally impaired extremity is evaluated. Muscle strength, the interval for both active and passive movements of the affected size were also assessed. Palpation of the humeral head at the posterior side of the shoulder is performed to evaluate the joint incongruence. In addition, we assess the limited external rotation of the shoulder and the presence of the Putti sign. While the shoulder is passively adducted and externally rotated with the elbow in 90 degrees of flexion, there is an elevation of the upper corner of the scapula termed as the Putti sign [35].

The modified Mallet's classification is used to compare preoperative and postoperative results. This classification includes five criteria: the ability to actively abduct the arm, external rotation of the arm, bring the hand behind the neck and over the mouth. Grade I indicates a firm shoulder or a flailing arm. Grade II indicates active abduction <30 degrees, no active external rotation, and the inability to bring the hand behind the neck and the back. The hand is brought to the mouth with the arm in abduction (the trumpeter sign). Grade III indicates active abduction of 30–90 degrees°, active external rotation <20 degrees, and difficulty placing the hand behind the neck and cephalad to the sacrum. There is still the trumpeter sign. Grade IV indicates active abduction >90 degrees, active external rotation >20 degrees, and no difficulty in bringing the hand behind the neck and over the thoracolumbar region of the back. The hand can be brought to the mouth, and there is no trumpeter sign. Grade V indicates a clinically normal shoulder. If a patient does not meet all five criteria for a grade, he or she is assigned a lower grade [35].

Antero-posterior radiographs of both shoulders must be taken to investigate the size (hypoplastic), location (elevated) of the scapula on the affected side. Moreover, the relationship between acromion and coracoid process, any change in glenoid are also assessed. It is possible to see the hypoplasia of the clavicle and the small proximal humeral epiphysis. The height of space between the acromion and humeral head may be longer than the normal side; the humerus may be more subtle or thicker according to metaphyseal and diaphyseal areas, and the length of the humeral shaft may be shorter [28]. Measurements of humeral retroversion can be done by magnetic resonance imaging or computed tomography (CT) scanning combined with the topographic location of the anterior crease of the elbow pointed upward [36, 37]. These two parameters are helpful techniques to get a more accurate grade of alignment for osteotomies to restore the plane of movement [38].

## 4. Glenoid anteversion osteotomy combined with tendon transfer

This technique was inspired by the hip's developmental dysplasia; the open reduction and soft tissue procedures are not always sufficient to maintain concentric hip joint reduction and acetabular osteotomies are sometimes necessary [39]. Severe cases of glenohumeral deformity, anteversion of the glenoid would contribute to the stability of an open joint reduction. Glenoidal osteotomy for anteversion

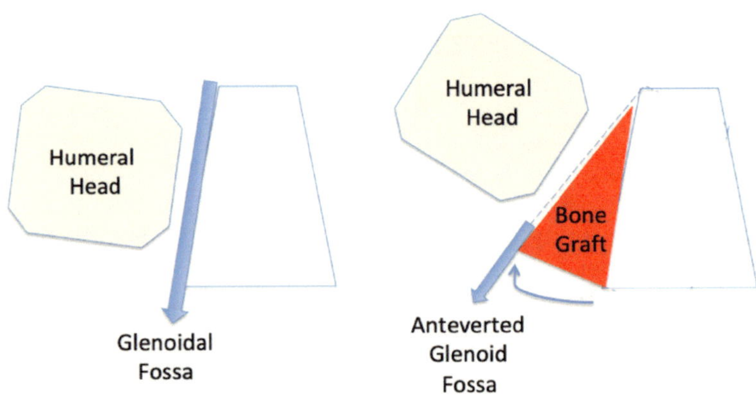


**Figure 2.**
*Osteotomy was performed with the protection of an intact anterior cortex to use as a hinge point, and bone graft was placed with the appropriate size.*

is performed to improve the glenoid retroversion whit taking the hinge point as an anterior cortex (**Figure 2**). When combined with a subscapularis slide and transfer of the teres major and latissimus dorsi, anteversion glenoid osteotomy and joint reduction would permit functional recovery of external shoulder rotation. Dodwell et al. [40] reported that they performed on 32 patients with severe glenohumeral dysplasia. Glenoidal osteotomy provided maintenance of the reduction of joint and functional improvement in the short term.

## 5. Humeral centering osteotomy

The humeral head centering osteotomy increases shoulder stabilization and resolves the anterior contractures with the subscapularis tenotomy. When humeral positioning becomes anatomical, the articular congruency can be adjusted and improve the motion arch of the shoulder. As in developmental hip dysplasia, the idea's origin is to reduce the joint centrally so that its normal growing process occurs. The articular reduction is provided with a medial derotational humeral osteotomy. Unfortunately, there is no standardized degree for angular derotational osteotomy. The ideal one is; first, the shoulder articulation is reduced with the external rotation maneuver. The humeral osteotomy is performed between insertion points of deltoid and pectoralis major muscles. and internally rotated until the patient's hand is brought over his or her abdomen (**Figure 3**). This procedure increases the anteversion of the humerus.

The indications for that procedure are:

- Posterior incongruence of the humeral head that causes dislocation,
- Age < 9 years
- The contraindications are:
- Active infection at the time of the surgery
- No active flexion of the elbow
- Deformity in the extension of the elbow

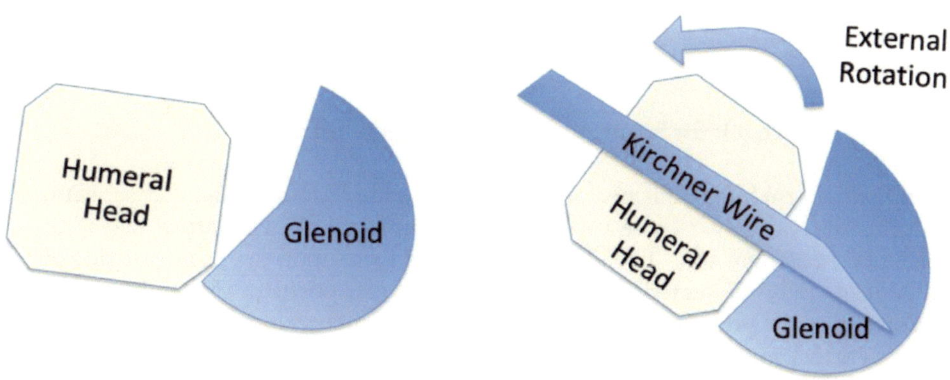


**Figure 3.**
*External rotation of humerus was performed to achieve glenohumeral joint reduction, and a Kirchner wire was placed for the temporary fixation.*

- Total brachial plexus lesion
- Trauma or infection sequel that destructs the articular surface
- Age > 9 years

For this procedure, a deltopectoral approach is performed. The subscapularis tenotomy with the anterior capsule is performed at the level of the lesser tuberosity to reach the joint. The reduction of the humeral head is rotated externally to reduce the joint. If there are difficulties or insufficiency for external rotation of the humerus, partial pectoralis major tenotomy can be made. There is no need for any tendon transfer. The humeral head is fixed and centered with a transarticular Kirschner wire. A transverse osteotomy of the humerus between the insertions of the deltoid and the pectoralis major muscles is performed. The humerus is internally rotated until the patient's hand is positioned over his abdomen, and then the osteotomy is fixed with a plate [35]. Vilaça et al. [35] reported 14 patients with centering osteotomy, and in all patients except one, shoulder dislocation to the posterior side could not be corrected.

## 6. Humeral external rotation osteotomy

Humeral external rotation osteotomy has been described by many surgeons [28, 30, 41–43]. It is mostly suggested for older children with advanced shoulder deformities. The aim of osteotomy is to increase the motion arch of external rotation of the affected shoulder. This osteotomy is accepted as standard treatment for late brachial plexus injury in older children. The results of this osteotomy have satisfactory results with an increase of both external rotation and abduction of the shoulder. Improvement of abduction is dependent on the improvement of the mechanical axis of the deltoid tendons. Moreover, surgeons keep in mind that there is always the possibility of the impairment of internal rotation with this technique. The osteotomy is usually performed proximal to the deltoid tuberosity level to improve the deltoid alignment (**Figure 4**). Some authors have suggested adding a flexion component to osteotomy distally to provide more elevation of the arm [42].

On the other hand, some others also have suggested adding a varus component to osteotomy to restore the abduction contracture [30]. If the plates and screws are used to fix osteotomy, there is no need for immobilization supplied externally by the cast splint. Several different approaches and levels have been described for the external rotational osteotomy of the humerus in literature. We will discuss them below.

### 6.1 Medial approach for humeral derotational osteotomy

A medial arm incision is performed along the medial intermuscular septum, and The interval between the anterior and posterior arm musculature is used to reach the osteotomy area. The ulnar nerve is just located on the posterior side of the septum and is dissected. The ulnar nerve is a transposition of the ulnar nerve performed to the posterior. In the anterior compartment, the median nerve and brachial artery are palpated and reflected with the biceps and brachialis muscle. The inter-muscular septum is followed through the medial aspect of the humerus and excised.

There are some advantages: Firstly, the scar is more cosmetic because the incision is located at the medial side of the arm and is difficult to see. The incision

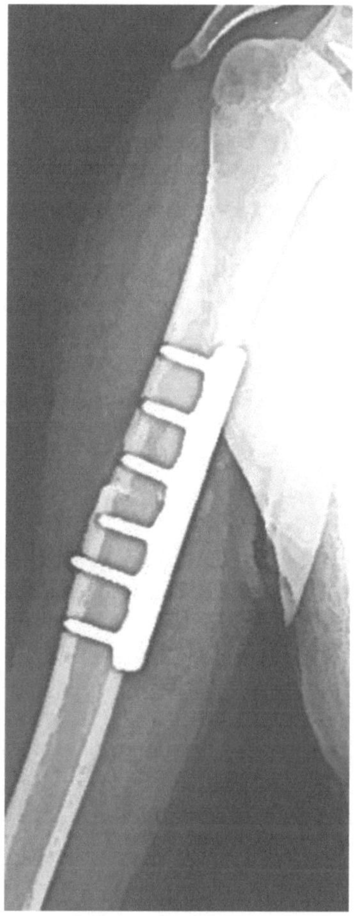

**Figure 4.**
*External rotational osteotomy at the level of deltoid tubercle just distal to the insertion point of the deltoid muscle. Osteotomy was fixed with a plate and screws.*

heals better compared to the lateral side. Arm positioning of the arm is easier after external derotational osteotomy places the arm onto the table, making internal fixation easier. In addition, plate application is more suitable at the anteromedial side of the humerus because of its anatomical shape. The disadvantage of the technique is related to its anatomy closer to neurovascular structures. The surgical anatomy is more dangerous because of the close relationship to nerves and is less familiar for the orthopedic surgeon [44].

## 6.2 Anterior approach for proximal humeral derotational osteotomy

An anterior incision is made through the interval between the biceps brachia and anterior part of the deltoid muscles to reach the proximal part of the humerus. Next, the insertion points of the subscapularis and pectoralis major muscles to humerus are identified. Then using the drill motor, holes through the line of osteotomy planned are opened, but at this phase, the osteotomy is not completed which is not completed. Next, the degree of external rotation of the distal part of the humerus is decided according to the hand position; if the hand can be touched the mouth, rotation of the humerus is enough. After completion of the osteotomy, the proximal and distal sides of the osteotomy are fixated. The use of highly strong sutures in the periosteum can be enough for stabilization if fragments are well impacted and stabilized. Otherwise, the osteotomy site is stabilized with generally one staple, but if the fixation is not unstable, the surgeon can use two staples [28].

The specific indications for this technique are

- Unimprovable internal rotation of shoulder accompanying to impairment in the function of the teres major and latissimus dorsi muscle in 4–8 years old
- Recrudesce in the dislocation of humerus head or the deformity of the affected side of the arm following a soft-tissue procedure in 4–8 years old
- Internal rotation deformity that can not be restored with procedures other than surgery or decline in the range of active motion through the external side in >8 years old

There are some advantages:

- The osteotomy site consists of a metaphyseal area (cancellous bone). Thus consolidation in there is quicker than other parts of the humerus.
- The staples that are used for fixation of the osteotomized bone are primary, simple devices. Therefore minimal distraction of periosteum and soft tissue is enough
- The osteotomy of the humerus and external rotation of distal part displace the insertion sides of the deltoid (makes tendons more strengthful) and pectoralis major muscle (increase in motion range of internal rotation) more lateral.

### 6.3 Humeral internal derotational osteotomy

Internal derotation osteotomy of the humerus is performed less often, and there has rarely been reported in the literature [45, 46]. It is described in young children who develop posterior dislocation of the shoulder early in the disease. The internal rotation osteotomy is performed for the reduction of the glenohumeral joint. However, this osteotomy is likely to result in more loss of external rotation. Releasing the internal rotator's muscles and the anterior capsule has to be added to improve the external rotation of the shoulder in these children. In addition, there may be necessary for the transfer of internal rotators to function as external rotators. Skibinski et al. [45] described internal rotation osteotomy (IRO) with a tendon transfer. They first performed soft tissue procedures and then tested the range of motion. Suppose the humeral head was dislocated while internal rotation, the internal humeral rotation was performed to strengthen the joint stability. They reported that the dynamic range of internal rotation difference in children treated with IRO was significantly higher than those treated without osteotomy. The other movements (including external rotation) were similar pre- and postop surgery in both groups. The authors concluded that the addition of IRO to soft tissue procedures improves internal rotation and maintains stable reduction without compromising other movements. Similarly, Kambhampati et al. [46] reported 183 cases of subluxation (101) and dislocation (82) of the shoulder secondary to obstetric brachial plexus palsy. The authors performed anterior release and reduction, and then they measured the degree of retroversion. They performed IRO if the humerus was retroverted more than 40 degrees° or if the head was volatile after reduction.

### 6.4 Humeral rotational osteotomy with lengthening over a nail

All the techniques that described derotational osteotomy of the humerus in the late treatment of OBPP have neglected upper limb length discrepancy, which is another sequel of OBPP. This technique represents the late treatment of OBPP in patients with upper limb length discrepancy, using derotational osteotomy and lengthening with an elongation nail. A standard deltopectoral approach was applied. Transverse osteotomy between the insertion of the deltoid and pectoralis major muscles was performed. Before the distal locking of the nail, adequate rotation of the humerus was decided intraoperatively by ascertaining that the ipsilateral hand could be placed to the mouth while putting the flexed elbow to the side of the trunk. Once the desired rotation was achieved, the distal locking screws were placed (**Figure 5**) [47].

This technique has some advantages: First, the elimination of length discrepancy improves the upper limb function by re-orientation of the shoulder arc into a more functional range. In addition, the appearance of the upper limb can be improved by visible antecubital fossa and diminished forearm pronation. Secondly, lengthening the humerus with the osteotomy above the deltoid insertion can lead to a more lateralized deltoid insertion, thus improving shoulder abduction more than expected. The disadvantages of this procedure are that it is impossible to add varus or flexion to the distal part of the humerus due to the use of the intramedullary elongation nail. Because ERO with added flexion to the distal part of the humerus to create increased flexion of the arm and adding a varus component to repair the abduction contracture is suggested in the literature [30, 42, 48]. We reported one patient with three years of follow-up. First, the proximal side of the osteotomy migrated the upper part at the end of 5 cm lengthening (**Figure 6**).

That problem could lead to restriction of shoulder motion. However, at the three years, Mallet score was four, and the patient was able to reach the occiput without any trumpet sign, and the palm rather than the dorsum was facing the mouth, which he could not do before the operation (**Figure 7**).

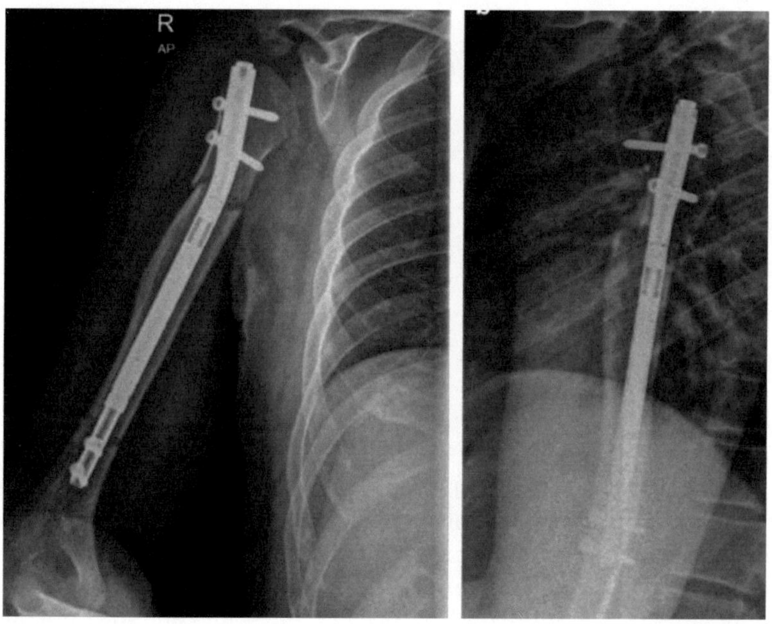


**Figure 5.**
*Postoperative plain AP and Lat. X-rays.*

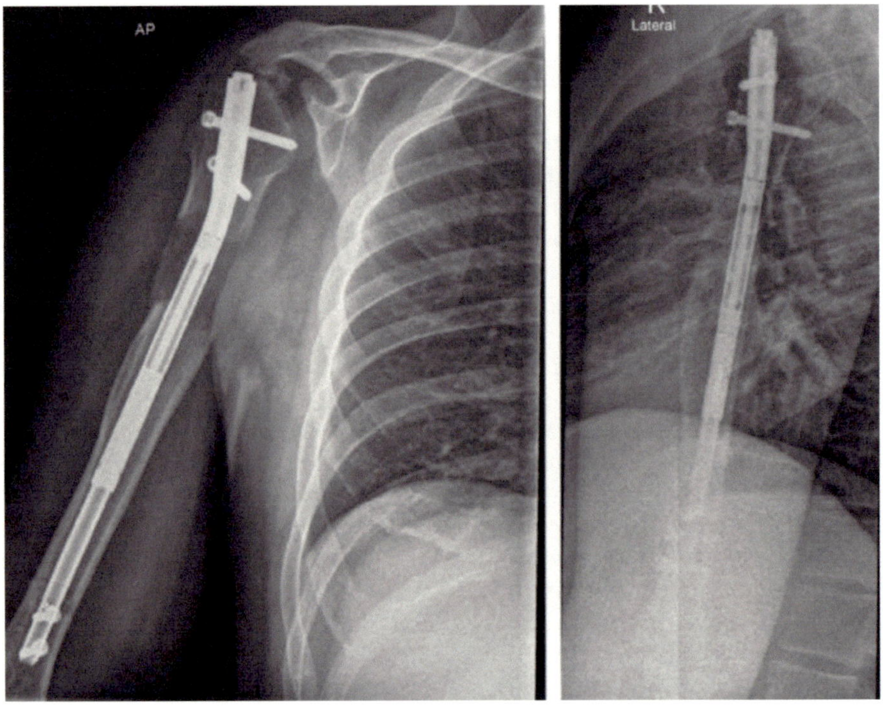


**Figure 6.**
*At the end of 5 cm distraction, AP and Lat. X-rays.*

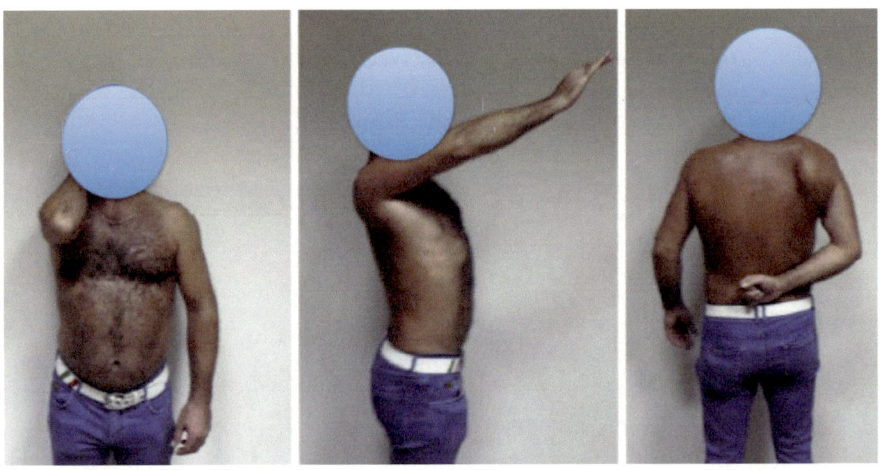

**Figure 7.**
*Range of motions at 36 months.*

## 6.5 Percutaneous humeral derotational osteotomy

The traditional humeral external derotation osteotomy method is open surgery and fixation with implants such as plates and nails. Open surgery often leaves a flagrant incision scar, but it can be hidden via a medial approach. Sometimes, other complications are resourced from implants, such as irritative effects, non-union, failure of implants, or peri-implant fracture [29, 30, 42]. When the implant has to be removed, it can be difficult, especially in the medial approach due to closer location to neurovascular structures. Therefore to avoid these complications, percutaneous osteot¬omy of the humerus and external fixation is designed. In the first step, two pins are placed at the level of the distal half of the deltoid muscle and below the proximal humeral physis through the lateral side of the humerus. Then, another two pins are placed at the distal insertion point of the deltoid muscle but more anteriorly than before two pins to provide interval while external rotating of the distal fragment of the humerus. The position of these two pins on the anterior plane is decided according to how much rotation is required. The second phase is performing the percutaneous transverse osteotomy of the humerus. The third phase is that the distal fragment is rotated externally till all pins are arranged in the same plane. One or two rods are used to connect the proximal and distal pins and stabilize the osteotomized bone [49]. Advantages of these techniques are

- Incision is minimal. Thus the development of scars does not cause cosmetic problems.

- The placement of the proximal side pins is distal to the deltoid, where there is no risk for physical bone and axillary nerve injuries [50]. In addition, the distal pins are located anteriorly away from the lateral side, where the radial nerve passes through the bone.

- Rotational control of the distal humerus is difficult during open reduction and plate fixation. However, in this technique, distal pins supply stability and controlling the distal fragment efficiently.

Aly et al. [49] reported that six cases that healing processes were completed at an average of 1–2 months without complication. In addition that they showed improvement in the shoulder motion.

## 7. Osteotomy of the radius and ulna or one-bone forearm

Mild rigid supination deformities can be treated with osteotomy of the radius or ulna [51]. However, osteotomy of both bones requires correcting severe supination deformities completely. Nowadays, the creation of one-bone forearm procedures is preferred to combined osteotomies for severe fixed supination deformities due to the recurrence overtime after combined osteotomies caused by persistent muscle imbalance and the ability to correct substantial deformities. A curvilinear incision is made along the distal radius and proximal ulna. The osteotomies are planned with the radius osteotomy 1 to 2 cm distal to the ulnar osteotomy. The interosseous membrane is incised to allow the radius to be positioned on top of the proximal ulna. The radius is manually mobilized toward the proximal ulna. The bones are coapted, the radius is rotated into the desired position, the plate is placed to the distal radius to connect to the proximal ulna [52].

## 8. Outcomes

Activities that require external rotation can be done quickly with humeral derotational osteotomy. Before surgery, many patients cannot perform self-care activities, such as eating, dressing, and washing. After surgery, most patients can dress, wash, perform self-cleaning, and eat themselves better and no longer need help. The Mallet score for shoulder function increases after osteotomy. The level of osteotomy is still controversial. Theoretically, rotational osteotomy between the insertions of the subscapularis and pectoralis major muscles improves the deltoid function. There are no standard methods of fixation. Osteotomy stabilization has varied from flimsy catgut sutures to rigid plates and screws. The fixation technique will affect postoperative rehabilitation. The improved outcome has been represented regardless of fixation [28–30].

## 9. Conclusion

The arm's fixed adduction and internal rotation are the most common deformities of the extremity in patients with a. In addition, the limited flexion-extension motion of the elbow because of fixed pronation of the forearm can be seen in brachial plexus birth injury. The surgical procedures performed to correct the shoulder deformity provide the range of motion to more acceptable mobility and position and are highly possible to affect the useability of all parts of the upper extremity. This is mostly seen in the patients with the latissimus dorsi and teres major muscles problems and abnormal radiographic findings of the glenohumeral joint. Difficulties in bringing the hand to the mouth without leaning the head forward and toward the involved side and incompetent abduction-flexion of the shoulder if the fixed internal rotation deformity of the shoulder is more than 20 degrees [53]. Suppose external rotation of the shoulder is less than 65 degrees and limited abduction at 80 degrees. In that case, it is impossible to reach the mouth by hand, significantly if the motion range of the hand wrist and elbow is impaired [54]. The soft-tissue contracture is released to improve the cosmetic appearance. Besides, the function of the joint improves slightly. However, there is an increase in only external rotation, not an increase in abduction is observed, and there is a high possibility for anterior dislocation of the shoulder. In addition, recurrence of the fixed internal rotation deformity reduces the range of rotational movement with time passing [53]. Sever described a technique that involves the release and replacement of the teres major and latissimus dorsi muscles to the posterior and lateral parts of the humerus to function as external rotators of the shoulder if muscle strength is enough. The glenohumeral joint has any abnormalities [20]. The osteotomy of the proximal humerus for the late treatment of brachial plexus birth injuries' suggested first time by Roger [21].

Since then, several techniques have been described, including either the proximal or the distal humeral derotational osteotomy in case of structural abnormality (irreducible internal rotation) and anatomical pathology (flattened humeral head or posterior subluxation) of the shoulder [14, 21, 32, 33, 53]. There is a gradual increase in the arc of active motion at the expense of passive motion. Therefore, rotation of the extremity can be increased during the growth of the extremity in a neutral position and alignment. This can result in changing the relationship between the joint congruency and the soft tissues that cover the joint. Therefore, surgeons must consider the alteration of the congruency due to the growth of the bones and soft tissues and not overcorrect the abnormality.

## Author details

Ahmet Emrah Açan[1*] and Ertuğrul Şahin[2]

1 Department of Orthopaedics and Traumatology, Faculty of Medicine, Balikesir University, Balıkesir, Turkey

2 Department of Orthopaedics and Traumatology, İzmir Kemalpaşa State Hospital, Izmir, Turkey

*Address all correspondence to: dremrahacan@hotmail.com

## References

[1] Sjoberg I, Erichs K, Bjerre I. Cause and effect of obstetric (neonatal) brachial plexus palsy. Acta Paediatr Scand. 1988;77(3):357-364.

[2] Sever JW. Obstetric Paralysis-Its Cause and Treatment. Can Med Assoc J. 1920;10(2):141-161.

[3] Strömbeck C, Krumlinde-Sundholm L, Forssberg H. Functional outcome at 5 years in children with obstetrical brachial plexus palsy with and without microsurgical reconstruction. Dev Med Child Neurol. 2000;

[4] Badger B. Perinatally acquired brachial plexus palsy - A persisting challenge. Acta Paediatr Int J Paediatr. 1997;86(11):1214-1219.

[5] Pondaag W, Malessy MJA, Van Dijk JG, Thomeer RTWM. Natural history of obstetric brachial plexus palsy: A systematic review. Dev Med Child Neurol. 2004;46(2):138-144.

[6] Kozin SH. Correlation between External Rotation of the Glenohumeral Joint and Deformity after Brachial Plexus Birth Palsy. J Pediatr Orthop. 2004;24:189-193.

[7] Pearl ML, Edgerton BW. Glenoid deformity secondary to brachial plexus birth palsy. J Bone Jt Surg - Ser A. 1998;80:659-667.

[8] Waters PM, Smith GR, Jaramillo D. Glenohumeral deformity secondary to brachial plexus birth palsy. J Bone Jt Surg - Ser A. 1998;80:668-677.

[9] Gudinchet F, Maeder P, Oberson JC, Schnyder P. Magnetic resonance imaging of the shoulder in children with brachial plexus birth palsy. Pediatr Radiol. 1995;25:125-128.

[10] van der Sluijs JA, van Ouwerkerk WJR, de Gast A, Wuisman PIJM, Nollet F, Manoliu RA. Deformities of the shoulder in infants younger than 12 months with an obstetric lesion of the brachial plexus. J Bone Jt Surg - Ser B. 2001;83:551-555.

[11] Moukoko D, Ezaki M, Wilkes D, Carter P. Posterior Shoulder Dislocation in Infants with Neonatal Brachial Plexus Palsy. J Bone Jt Surg - Ser A. 2004;86B:787-793.

[12] Troum S, Floyd WE, Waters PM. Posterior dislocation of the humeral head in infancy associated with obstetrical paralysis. A case report. J Bone Jt Surg - Ser A. 1993;75A: 1370-1375.

[13] Torode I, Donnan L. Posterior dislocation of the humeral head in association with obstetric paralysis. J Pediatr Orthop. 1998;18:611-615.

[14] Zancolli EA. Classification and management of the shoulder in birth palsy. Orthop Clin North Am. 1981;12:433-457.

[15] Pearl ML, Edgerton BW, Kon DS, Darakjian AB, Kosco AE, Kazimiroff PB, et al. Comparison of arthroscopic findings with magnetic resonance imaging and arthrography in children with glenohumeral deformities secondary to brachial plexus birth palsy. J Bone Jt Surg - Ser A. 2003;85A:890-898.

[16] Saifuddin A, Heffernan G, Birch R. Ultrasound diagnosis of shoulder congruity in chronic obstetric brachial plexus palsy. J Bone Joint Surg Br. 2002;84B:100-103.

[17] Zancolli EA ZE. Congenital brachial plexus exploration. In: Gupta A KS, LR S, editors. The Growing hand. London: Mosby; 2000. p. 805-823.

[18] Kennedy R. Suture of the brachial plexus in birth paralysis of the upper

extremity. Br Med J. 1903;1(2197): 298-301.

[19] HAT F. BIRTH PALSY : SUBLUXATION OF THE SHOULDER-JOINT IN INFANTS AND YOUNG CHILDREN. Lancet. 1913;3(1): 1217-1223.

[20] L'Episcopo J. Restoration of muscle balance in the treatment of obstetrical paralysis. New York Med J. 1939;39:357-363.

[21] Rogers MH. An Operation for the Correction of the Deformity Due to Obstetrical Paralysis. Bost Med Surg J. 1916;174:163-164.

[22] Pearl ML. Arthroscopic release of shoulder contracture secondary to birth palsy: An early report on findings and surgical technique. Arthrosc - J Arthrosc Relat Surg. 2003;19:577-582.

[23] Hui JHP, Torode IP. Changing glenoid version after open reduction of shoulders in children with obstetric brachial plexus palsy. J Pediatr Orthop. 2003;23:109-113.

[24] Pedowitz DI, Gibson B, Williams GR, Kozin SH. Arthroscopic treatment of posterior glenohumeral joint subluxation secondary to brachial plexus birth palsy. J Shoulder Elb Surg. 2007;16:6-13.

[25] Kozin SH, Chafetz RS, Barus D, Filippone L. Magnetic resonance imaging and clinical findings before and after tendon transfers about the shoulder in children with residual brachial plexus birth palsy. J Shoulder Elb Surg. 2006;15:554-561.

[26] Waters PM, Bae DS. Effect of tendon transfers and extra-articular soft-tissue balancing on glenohumeral development in brachial plexus birth palsy. J Bone Jt Surg - Ser A. 2005;87: 320-325.

[27] Pagnotta A, Haerle M, Gilbert A. Long-term results on abduction and external rotation of the shoulder after latissimus dorsi transfer for sequelae of obstetric palsy. Clin Orthop Relat Res. 2004;426:199-205.

[28] Kirkos JM, Papadopoulos IA. Late treatment of brachial plexus palsy secondary to birth injuries: Rotational osteotomy of the proximal part of the humerus. J Bone Jt Surg - Ser A. 1998;80:1477-1483.

[29] Al-Qattan MM. Rotation osteotomy of the humerus for Erb's palsy in children with humeral head deformity. J Hand Surg Am. 2002;27:479-483.

[30] Waters PM, Bae DS. The effect of derotational humeral osteotomy on global shoulder function in brachial plexus birth palsy. J Bone Jt Surg - Ser A. 2006;88:1035-1042.

[31] Zancolli EA, Zancolli ER. Palliative surgical procedures in sequelae of obstetric palsy. Hand Clin. 1988;4: 643-669.

[32] Glez Cuesta FJ, Lopez Prats F, Glez Lopez FJ, Bergada Sitja J. The role of bone operations as palliative surgical treatment for the sequelae of obstetrical brachial paralysis in the shoulder. Acta Orthop Belg. 1982;48:757-761.

[33] Goddard NJ, Fixsen JA. Rotation osteotomy of the humerus for birth injuries of the brachial plexus. J Bone Jt Surg - Ser B. 1984;66:257-259.

[34] Al Zahrani S. Modified rotational osteotomy of the humerus for Erb's palsy. Int Orthop. 1993;17:202-204.

[35] Vilaça PR, Uezumi MK, Zoppi Filho A. Centering osteotomy for treatment of posterior shoulder dislocation in obstetrical palsy. Orthop Traumatol Surg Res. 2012;98:199-205.

[36] Ivalde FC, Miguens GN, Socolovsky M. Using the main elbow

flexion skin crease as an intraoperative parameter to determine the degree of exorotation needed for humeral derotational osteotomies in upper-type brachial plexus patients. J Orthop Surg. 2018;26(3):230949901879271.

[37] Pearl ML, Batch M, Van De Bunt F. Humeral retroversion in children with shoulder internal rotation contractures secondary to upper-trunk neonatal brachial plexus palsy. J Bone Jt Surg - Am Vol. 2016;98(23):1988-1995.

[38] Itamura JM, Papadakis SA, Vaishnav S, Gourmet R. The relationship between main elbow flexion skin crease and osseous anatomy of the elbow joint. Surg Radiol Anat. 2009;31(1):55-58.

[39] Vitale MG, Skaggs DL. Developmental dysplasia of the hip from six months to four years of age. J Am Acad Orthop Surg. 2001;9(6):401-411.

[40] Dodwell E, O'Callaghan J, Anthony A, Jellicoe P, Shah M, Curtis C, et al. Combined glenoid anteversion osteotomy and tendon transfers for brachial plexus birth palsy: Early outcomes. J Bone Jt Surg - Ser A. 2012;94:2145-2152.

[41] Abzug JM, Chafetz S, Gaughan JP, Ashworth S, Kozin SH. Shoulder function after medial approach and derotational humeral osteotomy in patients with brachial plexus birth palsy. J Pediatr Orthop. 2010;30(5):469-474.

[42] Al-Zahrani S. Combined sever's release of the shoulder and osteotomy of the humerus for ERB's palsy. J Hand Surg Eur Vol. 1997;22:591-593.

[43] Al-Qattan MM, Al-Husainan H, Al-Otaibi A, El-Sharkawy MS. Long-term results of low rotation humeral osteotomy in children with erb's obstetric brachial plexus palsy. J Hand Surg Eur Vol. 2009;34(4):486-492.

[44] Kozin SH. Medial Approach for Humeral Rotational Osteotomy in Children with Residual Brachial Plexus Birth Palsy. Oper Tech Orthop. 2007;17(2):88-93.

[45] Sibiński M, Synder M. Soft tissue rebalancing procedures with and without internal rotation osteotomy for shoulder deformity in children with persistent obstetric brachial plexus palsy. Arch Orthop Trauma Surg. 2010;130(12):1499-1504.

[46] Kambhampati SBS, Birch R, Cobiella C, Chen L. Posterior subluxation and dislocation of the shoulder in obstetric brachial plexus palsy. J Bone Jt Surg - Ser B. 2006;88:213-219.

[47] Acan AE, Gursan O, Demirkiran ND, Havitcioglu H. Late treatment of obstetrical brachial plexus palsy by humeral rotational osteotomy and lengthening with an intramedullary elongation nail. Acta Orthop Traumatol Turc. 2018;52:75-80.

[48] Bae DS, Waters PM. External rotation humeral osteotomy for brachial plexus birth palsy. Tech Hand Up Extrem Surg. 2007;11(1):8-14.

[49] Aly A, Bahm J, Schuind F. Percutaneous humeral derotational osteotomy in obstetrical brachial plexus palsy: A new technique. J Hand Surg Eur Vol. 2014;39(5):549-552.

[50] Klepps S, Auerbach J, Calhon O, Lin J, Cleeman E, Flatow E. A cadaveric study on the anatomy of the deltoid insertion and its relationship to the deltopectoral approach to the proximal humerus. J Shoulder Elb Surg. 2004;13(322-7).

[51] Kozin SH. Treatment of the supination deformity in the pediatric brachial plexus patient. Tech Hand Up Extrem Surg. 2006;10:87-95.

[52] Sarah Ashworth SHK. Brachial Plexus Birth Palsy: Secondary Procedures to Enhance Function. In: Abzug, Joshua M., Scott H., Kozin, Zlotolow DA, editor. The Pediatric Upper Extremity. Springer; 2015. p. 1830-1831.

[53] WICKSTROM J, HASLAM ET, HUTCHINSON RH. The surgical management of residual deformities of the shoulder following birth injuries of the brachial plexus. J Bone Joint Surg Am. 1955;37:27-36.

[54] WICKSTROM J. Birth injuries of the brachial plexus. Treatment of defects in the shoulder. Clin Orthop. 1962;23: 187-196.

Section 3

# Non Operative Treatment

Chapter 5

# The Role of Functional Electrical Stimulation in Brachial Plexus Injury Repair

*Lin Yang, Yaxuan Li, Qianling Zhang, Mengnan Jiang and Jia He*

## Abstract

Brachial plexus injury (BPI) is a type of peripheral nerve injury, which is mainly manifested as upper limb sensory and motor dysfunction. Although the injury will not endanger life, it can cause serious functional loss and high disability rate, and eventually lead to patients unable to live normally. At present, the treatment methods for BPI mainly include conservative treatment, such as limb massage, exercise, drug therapy, autonomous movement and strength training; In clinic, nerve repair, nerve transplantation and muscle transfer can also be used. Although surgical treatment can better restore the function of injured brachial plexus, there is a certain risk, so it is not the first choice of treatment. As a mature electrical stimulation method, functional electrical stimulation (FES) can play a good role in promoting injured nerve regeneration and preventing skeletal muscle denervation atrophy, so it can be widely used in the treatment and functional recovery of BPI. This article will review the research progress of FES in the treatment of BPI.

**Keywords:** brachial plexus injury, functional electrical stimulation, research progress, clinical application, mechanism of action

## 1. Introduction

Brachial plexus injury (BPI) is a common type of peripheral nerve injury. In addition to muscle paralysis, motor and skin sensory functions will decrease or disappear in its innervated area, which has a high disability rate. In recent years, with the continuous occurrence of excessive stretching and traffic accidents, the incidence of BPI has also become higher and higher. Although the progress of peripheral nerve surgery has significantly improved the treatment effect of BPI, scar will be produced at the nerve repair site, which will inevitably distort the contour of nerve pulse reaching the sensory and motor cortex, and eventually make the injured peripheral nerve unable to regenerate effectively. Some regenerated axons will not be able to reach the receptors affected by the scar interface, and other relatively normal axons will also be misled, so that they can only re-dominate the wrong scar sensory receptors or irreversibly degenerate receptors, which will lead to impaired sensory function of shoulder joint and upper limb with loss of muscle strength [1]. Therefore, it is particularly important to find an effective method to improve the dysfunction after BPI.

In 1961, American expert liberson [2] first proposed functional electrical stimulation (FES) therapy, which belongs to the category of neuromuscular electrical stimulation (NMES). FES is mainly based on the patient's condition to set up the program in advance, and place the electrode on one or more groups of muscles of the patient's affected limb, and then the paralyzed muscles will contract under the stimulation of a certain intensity of low-frequency pulse current, so as to induce muscle movement or simulate normal autonomous movement (such as upper limb grasping, lower limb walking and other functional activities) At the same time, the repeated movement pattern information can be transmitted to the central nervous system, forming excitement marks on the cortex, and ultimately can achieve the purpose of restoring muscle movement and enhancing balance ability [3]. In 2015, Elzinga et al. [4] found that nerve repair is needed after nerve injury. If the time of nerve repair is appropriately prolonged and FES is used to stimulate motor and sensory neurons for a long time, the speed of nerve growth can be improved, and nerve fibers can grow into the innervated skeletal muscle accurately along the direction of electric field. As one of the promising therapeutic technologies in the field of modern clinical rehabilitation, FES can be used to treat BPI, play the role of promoting regeneration of injured brachial plexus and preventing denervated atrophy of skeletal muscle.

## 2. Clinical anatomy of the brachial plexus

### 2.1 Composition of brachial plexus

The brachial plexus is a collection of most of the nerve fibers of the 5th-8th cervical nerve anterior branch and the 1st thoracic nerve anterior branch, usually composed of five roots, three stems, six strands and three bundles. The 5 nerve roots from the spinal cord exit the intervertebral foramen at the same time as they branch out the dorsal scapular nerve ($C_{4\text{-}5}$), the long thoracic nerve ($C_{5\text{-}7}$), and the phrenic nerve ($C_{3\text{-}5}$). The five nerve roots form the superior, middle and inferior trunks on the lateral edge of the anterior scalene muscle, among them, $C_{5\text{-}6}$ constitutes the superior trunk, $C_7$ independently constitutes the middle trunk, and $C_8$-$T_1$ constitutes the inferior trunk. Each trunk is divided into anterior and posterior divisions above or behind the clavicle. The anterior division of the upper and middle trunks synthesize the lateral cord, and the main branches are the lateral root of median nerve, musculocutaneous nerve and lateral pectoral nerve; the anterior division of the lower trunk synthesize the medial cord, and the main branches are the medial antebrachial cutaneous nerve, ulnar nerve and medial root of median nerve; the posterior division of the three trunks converges into the posterior cord, the main branches are the subscapular nerve, thoracodorsal nerve, axillary nerve and radial nerve. The three bundles enter the axillary and send out nerve branches, which mainly control the sensory and motor functions of the upper limbs, shoulder back and chest (**Figure 1**) [5].

### 2.2 Major neural injury and its clinical expressions

BPI can generally be divided into upper brachial plexus injury, lower brachial plexus injury and complete brachial plexus injury [6]. The main manifestations of upper brachial plexus injury are that the shoulder joint cannot be abducted, the elbow joint cannot be flexed, the upper limb cannot rotate internally and externally, and the radial sensory disturbance, but the finger movement is still normal; the

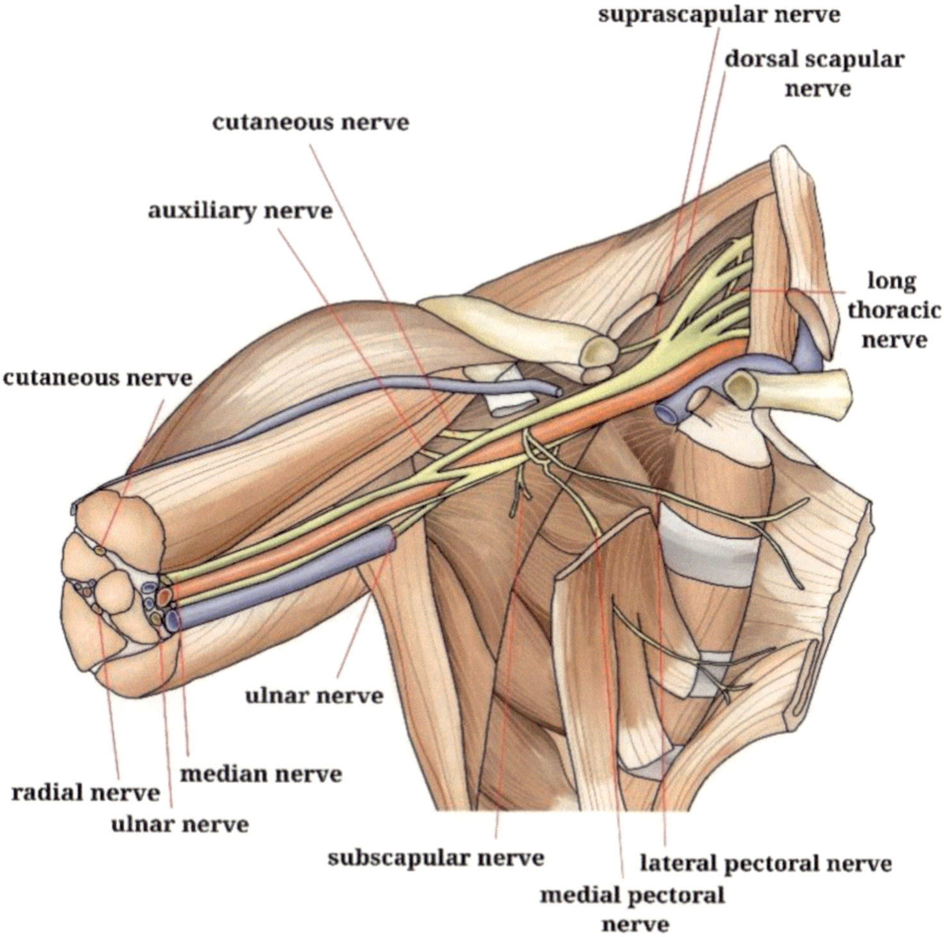


**Figure 1.**
*Anatomy of the course of the brachial plexus in the armpit (drawn by Jia He).*

main manifestations of lower brachial plexus injury were finger grasping dysfunction, sensory loss of ulnar skin of forearm and hand, but the activities of shoulder joint, elbow joint and wrist joint were normal; complete brachial plexus injury showed the disappearance of upper limb motor and sensory functions. The damage of different nerve branches also leads to the dysfunction of corresponding parts. For example, phrenic nerve injury can cause respiratory dysfunction, severe cases can cause apnea; musculocutaneous nerve injury can cause weakness in elbow flexion and weakened skin sensation on the outer forearm; axillary nerve injury mainly leads to deltoid muscle paralysis forming square shoulder; median nerve injury, as one of the common types of injury, is mainly manifested by the loss of sensory function on the radial side of the hand, forming "ape hand", as well as forearm pronation disorder; the main clinical manifestations of ulnar nerve injury is weakened wrist flexion ability and the distal end of the ring finger and little thumb cannot be flexed, resulting in the formation of "claw hand", which can also lead to loss of sensory function in the palm and the inner back of the hand; radial nerve injury mainly manifests as "wrist drop" caused by paralysis of the extensor muscle of the forearm, and accompanied by dorsal hand radial half and radial side of the two half finger proximal segment back skin sensory dysfunction (**Figure 2**).

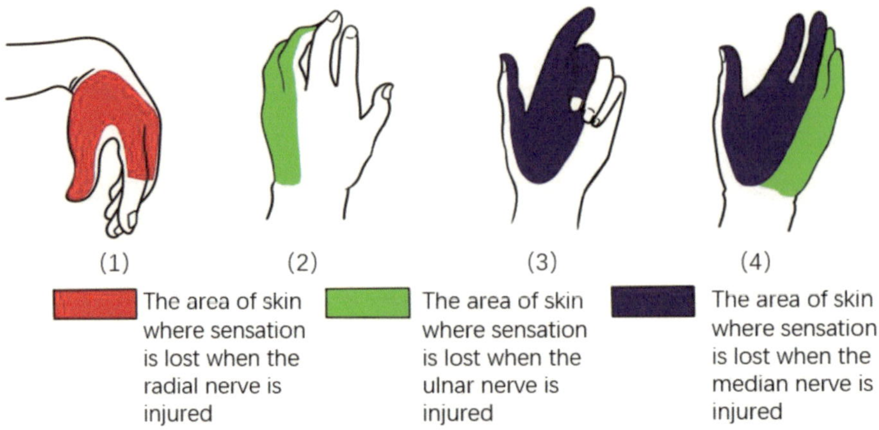


**Figure 2.**
*(1). Wrist drop (radial nerve injury); (2). "Claw hand" (ulnar nerve injury); (3). Median nerve injury in hand; (4). "Ape hand" (median nerve injury and ulnar nerve injury) (drawn by Jia He).*

## 3. Changes of regenerative microenvironment after brachial plexus injury

The repair process of BPI is related to many factors, such as the formation of regenerative microenvironment around the injury, the sprouting and extension of axons, the reinnervation of nerve to target tissue, axon regeneration and so on. The formation of regeneration microenvironment is an important factor affecting the repair of brachial plexus injury.

### 3.1 Establishment of nerve regeneration channels

After BPI, the axons and myelin sheath at the distal end of the injury degenerate and then disintegrate into nerve debris, Schwann cells (SCs) produce autophagy reaction, and eventually Wallerian degeneration occurs at the end of the nerve involved. In the early stage of injury, SCs can help macrophages to clear degenerative myelin debris, and the laminin secreted by it can form basement membranes to promote growth and provide channels, which can guide axons to grow rapidly in the right direction. The proliferating SCs form a solid cell cord (band of Büngner) in the nerve basal lamina enclosed by the basement membrane, which has a good guiding effect on the growth of nerve axons. The band of Büngner and nerve basal lamina can not only produce related molecules that promote axon regeneration, but also separate molecules that inhibit regeneration in the endoneurial tube, which can accelerate the regeneration and repair of injured nerve [7, 8].

### 3.2 Neurotrophic factor regulation

After BPI, SCs, nerve axons, fibroblasts and so on will produce a class of polypeptide called neurotrophic factors (NTFs), which have a variety of activities and can exert efficient physiological effects by binding to specific receptors on the surface of target cells [9]. It mainly includes 3 categories: ①. Neurotrophin, including nerve growth factor (NGF), brain-derived neurotrophin factor (BDNF), neurotrophin-3 (NT-3), neurotrophin-4/5 (NT-4/5), and neurotrophin-6 (NT-6), neurotrophin-7 (NT-7) derived from non-mammals, etc. ②. Neurocytokinin, including ciliary neurotrophic factor (CNTF), interleukin-1,3,6 (IL-1,3,6), etc. ③. Fibroblast growth factor (FGF), and other NTFs such as glial cell line-derived neurotrophic factor (GDNF), insulin like growth factor (IGF) and so on. These NTFs can play different roles in the regeneration and repair of injured brachial plexus, for example: ①. NGF combined with p75 can block p75 induced nerve cell death, thus can promote the intracellular signal transduction of injured nerve, which is conducive to accelerating the growth of axons and promoting the recovery of nerve function [10]. ②. The increased expression of BDNF and its tyrosine kinase receptor B (TrkB) mRNA can reshape synapses, restore neural pathways, and promote regeneration of axons and reconnection of injured muscles. ③. GDNF can nourish the axons and SCs of mature spinal cord, which is beneficial to axonal regeneration. It has been found that after sciatic nerve transection in rats, SCs can continuously express GDNF mRNA in nerve fibers for more than 5 months [11]. ④. Other studies have confirmed that NTFs can promote nerve cell regeneration and accelerate motor nerve conduction velocity to a certain extent [12].

### 3.3 Immune response

A series of immune responses after nerve injury can inhibit nerve regeneration and repair to a certain extent. The occurrence of immune response may be related to the following ways: ①. Nerve injury can destroy the blood-nerve barrier, resulting in the leakage of neurogenic antigens to nearby lymph nodes and the production of specific antibodies, which will enter the blood circulation and cause immune response. ②. There are antigen-presenting cells in the nerve tissue. After nerve injury, antigen-presenting cells can express MHC class II antigens on their cell membranes after ingesting neurological antigens, and are taken up by T cells in the nerves to produce an immune response. ③. After the antigen-presenting cells ingest neurogenic antigens, they can also be presented to T cells in the blood by intra-nerve microvascular endothelial cells to stimulate an immune response. The immune response will have a significant inhibitory effect on nerve regeneration and repair [13].

### 3.4 Inflammatory response

Wallerian degeneration occurs immediately after BPI. Within 24 hours after injury, SCs demyelinated by degrading myelin basic protein, and then macrophages migrated to the nerve injury through blood vessels [14]. During Wallerian degeneration, SCs and macrophages phagocytize the denatured myelin, which is conducive to nerve regeneration, and the occurrence of inflammatory reaction is mainly related to macrophages. Macrophages can participate in the phagocytosis of degenerated myelin, and secrete the active factor oncomodulin to promote the proliferation of SCs, thereby promoting axon regeneration. The glial cells activated at the nerve injury can secrete cytokines that promote or inhibit the inflammatory response, among which pro-inflammatory factors (such as IL-1, IL-2, IL −6 and tumor necrosis factor (TNF)), which are mainly produced in the first stage of Wallerian degeneration, and promote the recruitment of macrophages 2-3 days after nerve injury; while, anti-inflammatory factors (such as IL-10 and transforming growth factor β(TGF-β)) are produced after macrophage recruitment and attenuate the inflammatory response [15]. After BPI, SCs, macrophages, and mast cells can immediately produce endogenous TNF-α, and the rapidly increasing TNF-α in the lesion site can also recruit a large number of macrophages to swallow degeneration myelin. IL-1 is an important pro-inflammatory factor in the process of nerve injury, and its members include IL-1α, IL-1β and so on. After 5-6 hours of nerve injury, SCs that lose close contact with axons can quickly up-regulate IL-1α mRNA and IL-1α protein [16]. IL-1α can induce fibroblasts to accumulate in the injured area and produce IL-6. IL-6 can enhance T cell activity and act on SCs, and participate in the regeneration of peripheral nerves by up-regulating pro-inflammatory response genes and immune protease subunits [17].

### 3.5 Hormonal regulation

After BPI, progesterone, thyroid hormone, adrenocorticotropic hormone and so on can participate in the repair of damaged nerves. Progesterone not only promotes the sciatic nerve of damaged male rats, but also binds to receptors to regulate the expression of SCs [18]. Thyroid hormone can play an important role in the growth and development of the central nervous system and the repair of peripheral nerve damage. It can make non-nerve cells produce NTFs to promote axon repair and regeneration, and can also act on SCs to maintain neuronal activity and promote nerve growth [19]. Adrenocorticotropic hormone can accelerate the regeneration of axons, which is beneficial to promote the regeneration and repair of injured nerves [20].

## 4. Treatment of brachial plexus injury

The treatment methods used vary according to the injury site, injury type, injury severity, and time after injury. The purpose of treatment is to reduce permanent disability and restore or improve upper limb function. The mild cases may be temporarily observed, functional exercises shall be performed, and re-examination shall be carried out regularly, while the severe cases may require treatment such as surgery.

### 4.1 General conservative treatment

General conservative treatment mainly includes local physical therapy, acupuncture, massage, comprehensive rehabilitation exercise, standardized electrical stimulation therapy, oral neurotrophic drugs, etc. In order to promote the regeneration of injured brachial plexus and prevent skeletal muscle denervation atrophy, so as to ensure that joints and muscles can work normally and move in the normal range of activity.

### 4.2 Surgical treatment

At present, the commonly used clinical surgical treatment methods for BPI mainly include nerve repair, nerve transplantation, nerve suture, neurolysis, nerve transfer (neuralization), tendon/muscle transfer, free functional muscle transfer (FFMT) and so on [21]. (1). Nerve suture: For patients with sharp cuts or penetrating injuries, the musculocutaneous nerve, lateral spinal cord or superior nerve trunk can be sutured directly end-to-end. (2). Exo-plexus nerve transfer: ①. Spinal accessory nerve (SAN) transfer: SAN is well used for nerve transfer because it has sufficient length and motor axons. Up to 95% of BPI patients retain SAN, which can be widely transferred to different targets to restore storage functions [22]. ②. Intercostal nerves (ICNs) transfer: Seddon first described the ICNs transfer, which borrowed ulnar nerve transplantation to transfer ICNs to the musculocutaneous nerve (MCN ) to restore the elbow flexion function of patients with complete brachial plexus injury. Other surgeons may prefer to transfer the motor branches of ICNs directly to the biceps brachii branch of MCN to obtain more reliable motor function recovery [23]. ③. Contralateral $C_7$ nerve root transfer: It is the safest surgical method for the treatment of brachial plexus root avulsion [24]. (3). Iintra-plexus nerve transfer: ①. Triceps branch of radial nerve (TRN) transfer: Since TRN runs along the proximal end of the upper arm with the radial and axillary nerves, transplanting one of the branches to the other nerve will not affect the normal function of its innervated area. Therefore, TRN is often transferred to axillary nerve to treat shoulder pain, shoulder subluxation, hand abduction insufficiency and other clinical symptoms caused by axillary nerve injury [25]. ②. Double nerve transfer method (Mackinnon's method, Oberlin II method): Oberlin et al. [26] elbow flexion dysfunction caused by brachial plexus root avulsion can be treated by transferring some of the ulnar nerve bundle branches located in the upper arm to the biceps muscle branch of the musculocutaneous nerve. ③. Medial pectoral nerve (MPN) transfer: can be used to treat obstetric brachial plexus injury [27]. ④. Transfer of brachialis muscle branch of the musculocutaneous nerve: This method has a good therapeutic effect whether it is to reduce the neuropathic pain of patients with simple brachial plexus inferior trunk injury, or to restore the function of finger holding [28]. (4). Gracilis FFMT: The gracilis muscle is considered to be a good BPI muscle metastasis due to its reliable proximal neurovascular pedicle and long tendon length, which can be used to treat elbow flexion difficulties caused by complete brachial plexus injury [29].

## 5. Development of functional electrical stimulation

### 5.1 Selection of functional electrical stimulation methods

At present, due to different stimulation methods and electrode placement positions, there are three main stimulation modes of FES: surface electrical stimulation, percutaneous electrical stimulation, and fully implanted electrical stimulation [30]. Each method has both advantages and disadvantages. (1). The advantage of surface electrical stimulation is that there is no cumbersome operation of embedding the electrode in the body, and no need to perform secondary operations for removing and needle electrodes, which reduces the possibility of trauma. This method is convenient and does not cause pain, but also has a very wide range of indications. However, it has the following disadvantages: ①. The patient will feel discomfort when the stimulation intensity is high and there will be a risk of scalding the skin, so the stimulation intensity and stimulation depth will become relatively limited, which leads to the ineffective stimulation of deep muscles, so that the effect produced is not very ideal. ②. Since most of the surface stimulation must be performed in the hospital, this will cause the interval between two stimulations to be too long, and the patient's compliance will become worse. ③. Stimulating a single muscle will also affect the contraction and relaxation of surrounding muscles, reducing its specificity. (2). The advantages of percutaneous electrical stimulation is that it is relatively simple and easy to implement, and has a wide range of indications, but it cannot stimulate the wounded skin, and there may be adverse reactions such as infection or skin damage. (3). The advantages of fully implanted electrical stimulation: ①. It can not only stimulate for a long time, but also maintain a high selective stimulation in the case of low power, and the effect is reliable. ②.It can avoid skin infection and damage caused by percutaneous stimulation. ③. It can avoid the inconvenience and discomfort caused by surface stimulation, and can prevent the defects that cannot be accurately located due to low specificity [30]. However, the implanted electrode may also cause the electrode to shift or fall off, the battery is exhausted, the connection points between the electrodes are not firm and so on, which may cause complications such as infection of the electrode port and the body's rejection of the electrode [31].

### 5.2 Selection of functional electrical stimulation time

Electrical stimulation (ES) can promote injured nerve regeneration and functional recovery, but how to choose the best stimulation time is still controversial. Studies have shown that the immediate application of ES to the early injured nerve can accelerate axon regeneration and nerve function recovery [32], but this effect may only play in the initial stage of nerve regeneration, and will become smaller or even disappear after the beginning of nerve growth [33]. Some studies also believe that the above effects can also be achieved after a short delay in the FES start time [34]. The exact mechanism for the short-term delay of ES to accelerate neural recovery is still unclear, which may be related to the up-regulation of NGF expression by ES [35, 36]. As to whether ES can promote nerve regeneration at other time points after nerve injury, different researchers have put forward different opinions. For example, Zanakis [37] showed that once nerve regeneration starts, the presence or absence of electric field stimulation will not affect it. After animal experiments, Shen [38] found that FES can still promote nerve regeneration after 20 or even 60 days of nerve injury, and all the morphological, electrophysiological and neurological function indicators of peripheral nerves show a significant upward trend. For the stimulation of denervated muscles, it is generally believed that it should be performed immediately after denervation, in order to prevent muscle atrophy and restore motor function to the greatest extent.

### 5.3 Selection of functional electrical stimulation parameters

There are many factors that can affect the therapeutic effect of FES, and stimulation parameters are one of them. So we mainly discuss the settings of the following parameters. (1). Stimulation current: The commonly used stimulation currents in clinic mainly include electric field, electromagnetic field, intermediate frequency electrical stimulation, pulse electrical stimulation, constant weak direct current stimulation, etc. They can promote peripheral nerve repair, accelerate nerve fiber regeneration, and prevent muscle atrophy. (2). Stimulation intensity: Different intensities of es will have different effects on the regeneration of nerve fibers. For example, using 1 mA current to stimulate the injured nerve can significantly increase the nerve conduction speed, but the current intensity of 4 mA has a detrimental effect on regenerating nerve fibers [39]. For the stimulation of denervated muscles, due to the large amount of fat and connective tissue present in it, which have a strong current transfer ability, it can reduce the current reaching the muscle cells, so that muscle cells must be stimulated by high current or even exponential current to reach the excited state. (3). Stimulation pulse: The research found that the pulse used for stimulation can be divided into single-phase pulse and two-phase pulse. Because monophasic pulses apply energy to the body, and this energy will never be removed. Therefore, it may cause potential damage to the stimulated tissue, while biphasic pulses use pulses of different amplitudes alternately on the body surface Stimulation, which can significantly reduce the damage to the body [40]. In summary, the optimal parameters of FES have not yet been unified, and further research is still needed. At the same time, the effects of early, middle and late nerve recovery must be analyzed to achieve satisfactory results.

## 6. Application of functional electrical stimulation in brachial plexus injury

### 6.1 Localization effect of functional electrical stimulation in interscalene brachial plexus nerve block

Interscalene brachial plexus nerve block anesthesia is a common local nerve block anesthesia method in clinic, which is often used in the operation anesthesia of upper limb dysfunction caused by BPI. Traditional interscalene brachial plexus nerve block is mainly based on anatomical landmarks and the clinical experience of the anesthesiologist, and the success rate and effect are very different. In the process of anesthesia operation, blind detection of nerve position with puncture needle may lead to anesthesia failure, and patients may also have nerve injury phenomenon, which seriously affects the success rate and safety of Interscalene brachial plexus nerve block anesthesia. The use of neural electrical stimulator can optimize the above problems [41]. Zhao Xiaojuan et al. [42] 50 patients who needed upper limb surgery under Interscalene brachial plexus nerve block anesthesia into observation group and control group with 25 cases in each group. Before anesthesia, the two groups of patients were monitored by ECG, peripheral veins were opened, and midazolam 2 mg was administered intravenously. The patient was placed in a supine position, the affected limb was placed next to the trunk, and the head was tilted to the opposite side. The use of low-frequency ES can better increase the level of cAMP in nerve cells, thereby inducing cells to conduct synthetic reactions. This response can promote dorsal root ganglion (DRG) growth by up-regulating cell growth-related proteins and cytoskeleton proteins [43]. The initial current of the stimulator is set to 1.0 mA and the frequency is 1.0 Hz. When the puncture needle is close to the nerve trunk, it can cause the effect muscles innervated by the nerve to contract. Adjust the position of the stimulating needle to the median nerve or radial nerve or ulnar nerve of the patient's upper limbs. When the current is gradually reduced to 0.2-0.3 mA, there will be no effective muscle contraction. After confirming that there is no blood sucked back, inject 1% lidocaine into the extension tube connected to the insulated needle. In the control group, the traditional allosensory method was used for interscalene brachial plexus block. After observing various anesthesia indicators, it was found that the overall excellent and good rate of the observation group was higher than that of the control group, while the anesthesia operation time and the incidence of adverse reactions were significantly lower than that of the control group. It can be seen that the use of nerve stimulator to guide interscalene brachial plexus nerve block can significantly shorten the time of anesthesia, increase the success rate of anesthesia, and reduce the incidence of adverse reactions. It has very important clinical significance for upper limb surgery [44].

### 6.2 Rehabilitation effect of functional electrical stimulation in brachial plexus injury

After clinical practice, it was found that conventional conservative treatment combined with standardized electrical stimulation can achieve better rehabilitation effects. Standardized electrical stimulation therapy refers to the combination of low-frequency electrical stimulation and medium-frequency electrical stimulation, and then placing electrodes on the corresponding damaged muscles of the patient to promote the regeneration and repair of injured nerves and prevent denervation of skeletal muscles. At present, BPI comprehensive rehabilitation training takes many forms. For example, Liu Suzhe [45] randomly divided 100 children with obstetric brachial plexus palsy (OBPP) into two groups, one of which received routine rehabilitation (oral neurotrophic drugs, self-functional exercise at home, etc.), while the other group used a neuromuscular electrical stimulator on the basis of conventional rehabilitation treatment. The results showed that the addition of electromyographic stimulation can significantly improve the prognostic rate of children with affected limbs. Liu Hui [46] took 36 children who were treated for brachial plexus injury as the research object and were randomly divided into control group and experimental group, with 18 cases in each group. The control group was treated with acupuncture and the experimental group was combined with neuromuscular electrical stimulation on the basis of the control group. A comparative analysis of the treatment effects of the two groups of children found that the implementation of neuromuscular electrical stimulation combined with acupuncture therapy has a significant therapeutic effect and can effectively restore the function of the injured muscles of the children. Gu Yudong et al. [47] took 43 BPI patients admitted to their hospital as research subjects and randomly divided them into a treatment group and a control group. The 21 patients in the treatment group received comprehensive rehabilitation treatment such as percutaneous nerve stimulation and intermediate frequency electrotherapy. The control group did not take such treatment measures. The results of the study showed that compared with the observation group, the branch and total branch injury function scores of the treatment group were significantly higher than those of the control group, and the electromyography results showed that the receptor nerve regeneration potential appeared earlier in the treatment group. The above only exemplified part of the electrical stimulation combined with conventional rehabilitation training, and the results all show that such comprehensive therapy has played a better role in repairing brachial plexus injury. In addition, FES also has the characteristics of simple operation, safe and effective, no side effects and so on, it can be widely used in clinical practice.

### 6.3 Therapeutic effect of functional electrical stimulation on neuropathic pain caused by brachial plexus injury

In a prospective epidemiological survey, it was found that 60 of the 107 BPI patients who were diagnosed with neuropathic pain using the DH4 questionnaire were diagnosed. Neuropathic pain will have a certain impact on the patient's mind and quality of life [48]. At present, the commonly used clinical treatment measures are mainly to control symptoms by taking painkillers, but the results obtained are not optimistic, and there is a problem of treating the symptoms but not the root cause. Therefore, it is especially important to find a way to relieve or even eradicate neuralgia. Sun Yanli et al. [49] gave 31 patients with BPI combined with neuralgia to improve circulation, nutritional nerves, pain relief and other conventional treatments, and then supplemented with electrical stimulation (waveform: triangle wave, intensity: 20-30 mA, frequency: 50-100 Hz, pulse width: 10MS, time: 1 time/d, 30 min/time, 10 times as a course of treatment). After using the visual analogue scoring method, pain assessment form, and sleep self-rating scale to assess the degree of pain, it was found that after 3-4 electrical stimulation treatments, 93.5% of patients reported that it was effective, and the number and duration of burst pain were significantly reduced compared to before treatment. After 2 treatment cycles, all patients have reduced the use of painkillers to varying degrees, and 96.7% of patients have controlled their pain in an ideal state. This study shows that the use of FES can relieve neuropathic pain caused by BPI to a certain extent, and can improve the quality of life of patients.

## 7. Physiological mechanism of functional electrical stimulation for brachial plexus injury

The mechanism by which FES exerts the above effects is not clear, but a large number of studies have shown that it is closely related to factors such as promoting the secretion of SCs and NTFs, promoting axon regeneration, increasing blood supply, protecting muscle fibers, and reducing muscle fatigue.

### 7.1 Physiological mechanism of functional electrical stimulation promoting nerve regeneration

The electric field generated by ES can stimulate SCs to crawl, migrate, proliferate and divide [50], making them further secrete NTFs such as BDNF, NGF and NT 4 / 5 [51, 52]. Moreover, the electric field has a certain tendency to the structural proteins, microfilaments and microtubules of axons, which can not only improve the nerve growth speed, but also make the broken axons grow into the distal nerve stump along the correct direction [53]. When the axon enters the neural tube of the distal nerve stump, the number of axons passing through the repair site can be increased to promote the increase in the number of motor neurons, sensory neurons and the density of regenerative nerves [43], thus maximizing nerve function degree of recovery.

ES can increase the level of $Ca^{2+}$ by inducing cell membrane depolarization and opening voltage-gated calcium channels, and the increase of $Ca^{2+}$ can raise the expression of BDNF and its TrkB mRNA, which is most closely related to motor neuron regeneration [54], It can promote the reconnection of axons and muscles, accelerate nerve conduction speed and enhance muscle fiber vitality, and then restore damaged nerve function. Through research, it is found that the main target of ES in downstream pathways is cyclic adenosine monophosphate (cAMP). The use of low-frequency ES can better increase the level of cAMP in nerve cells and induce cells to undergo synthetic reactions, which can upregulate the expression of cells growth-related proteins and cytoskeleton proteins (including actin, tubulin, and growth-associated protein 43) [55] to promote Dorsal root ganglion (DRG) neurite outgrowth. At the same time, ES can also induce cAMP to activate phosphokinase A (PKA), and activated PKA can mediate the phosphorylation of cAMP response element binding protein (CREB) [56], which in turn activates downstream pathways and increases the expression of BDNF. When BNDF rises to a certain level, the continuous increase of cAMP can be maintained by inhibiting phosphodiesterase [57]. Therefore, as long as a short electrical stimulation can cause a series of closed-loop reactions that promote cAMP to rise and maintain a certain level.

### 7.2 Physiological mechanism of functional electrical stimulation inhibiting skeletal muscle atrophy

Using NMES to stimulate the damaged muscles can make the muscles contract passively and rhythmically, which can expand the nutritional blood vessels of the damaged brachial plexus. The increased blood flow and circulatory stretching caused by vasodilation may stimulate the production of vascular endothelial growth factor. These growth factors can reduce the rate of vascular degeneration and induce angiogenesis, which can accelerate the metabolism of denervated muscles, provide various nutritional factors required for nerve regeneration, and remove harmful substances to prevent them from accumulating in muscles [58], and will not affect the reinnervation of nerves, at the same time, it can accelerate the establishment of effective contact between axons and distal effectors, restore the ultrastructure of myofibrils and membrane $Ca^{2+}$ channels, thereby reducing muscle atrophy and improving muscle function [59]. There are also certain differences in the effects of different intensities of electrical stimulation on damaged muscles and the mechanism of action, For example, medium frequency electrotherapy is a positive and negative alternating current, which has no electrolytic effect on body tissues, there is no acid–base reaction under the electrode, which can prevent chemical irritation to the skin and reduce skin resistance. When the current intensity is high, the current can directly reach the deep tissues, and the distance between cells and tissues can be increased when used in the early stage of injury, thereby effectively preventing the adhesion of muscle fibers, tissue fibers and nerve fibers, and ultimately achieving significant relief of muscle pain and reduction the purpose of tissue adhesion and relieving scar contracture secondary to brachial plexus surgery [60]. High frequency electrical stimulation plays an important role in maintaining the contractile function of type II muscle fibers, reducing muscle fatigue and preventing muscle atrophy [61].

Over time, most patients with BPI will experience varying degrees of muscle atrophy, accompanied by programmed apoptosis of denervated skeletal muscle cells [62]. When muscle atrophy reaches a certain degree, new nerves will not be accepted and irreversible dysfunction will occur [63]. Paillard et al. [64] and others believe that ES can activate satellite cells and promote the expression of myoblast related biomarkers, which can reduce the expression of ubiquitin ligase gene related to muscle atrophy, so as to remodel muscle fibers. Honda et al. [65] found that muscle contraction induced by ES can prevent the reduction of muscle nucleus caused by apoptotic changes, thereby reducing the aggregation of macrophages. These changes may prevent the signal transduction of fibroblasts into myofibroblasts through the IL-1β/TGF-β1 pathway, thus achieving the goal of inhibiting muscle fibrosis and atrophy. FES can also induce mitochondrial generation, improve mitochondrial function and prevent mitochondrial enzyme inactivation, which can increase the energy supply of muscle cells and prevent rapid atrophy and apoptosis of skeletal muscle [47].

## 8. Conclusion

In recent years, with the frequent occurrence of accidental injuries such as car accidents, external force pulling, and heavy object crushing, BPI has shown an upward trend year by year. Mild cases may have temporary upper limb dysfunction with tingling or burning sensation and arm numbness and weakness; severe cases may have varying degrees of muscle paralysis or atrophy of upper limbs, accompanied by weakened or disappeared motor and sensory functions, and even appear complete loss of upper limb function. Therefore, repairing the damaged brachial plexus and promoting its functional recovery is an important problem that needs to be solved urgently. The solution of this problem is related to the establishment of nerve regeneration channels, neurotrophic factor regulation, immune response, inflammatory response, hormone regulation and other local micro The formation of the environment is closely related. At present, the commonly used clinical surgical treatment methods for BPI mainly include nerve transplantation, nerve suture, nerve transfer (neuralization), etc. However, after surgery, combined with conventional treatments such as FES can achieve a best rehabilitation effect. FES can play a role in all aspects of BPI treatment. For example, in the repair of brachial plexus injury, FES combined with ultrasound can accurately locate the nerve block site and shorten the anesthesia time; in the process of postoperative rehabilitation, combined with conventional conservative treatment can promote the regeneration of injured brachial plexus and inhibit denervated skeletal muscle atrophy. In addition, FES can relieve neuropathic pain caused by BPI.

Although FES has a certain promoting effect in the various processes of brachial plexus repair, each BPI patient's blood supply, degree of injury, psychological endurance and self-rehabilitation ability are different, and FES itself also has ①. Cost problem. ②. Electrode material selection. ③. Optimal combination of electrical stimulation parameters. ④. Optimal stimulus site selection and other problems have not been resolved, so the efficiency of functional recovery still cannot reach the inherent motor ability of human beings. Therefore, we hope that in future research, we can conduct in-depth studies on the adjustment of the frequency, amplitude, and pulse width of electrical stimulation, as well as at which stage of nerve repair to start electrical stimulation, so as to overcome the problems of nerve regeneration and nerve function repair.

## Acknowledgements

The completion of the chapter is attributed to many people's support and encouragement. First and foremost, I want to thank the Key Laboratory of Human-Machine-Intelligence Synergic System, Shenzhen Institutes of Advanced Technology, Chinese Academy of Sciences (Director, Professor Guang Lin Li), and Guangdong-Hong Kong-Macao Joint Laboratory of Human-Machine Intelligence-Synergy Systems.

Also, I would like to express my sincere gratitude to the fund supports of National Natural Science Foundation of China (Grant Nos. 81960419; 81760416 and 81927804) and also to. Last my thanks would go to my student, Ms. Zijun Zhang and Mr. Xinkuan Liao who search and collect references for the completion of this chapter.

## Nomenclature

| | |
|---|---|
| BPI | Brachial Plexus Injury |
| FES | Functional Electrical Stimulation |
| NMES | Neuromuscular Electrical Stimulation |
| SCs | Schwann Cells |
| NTFs | Neurotrophic Factors |
| NGF | Nerve Growth Factor |
| BDNF | Brain-Derived Neurotrophin Factor |
| NT | Neurotrophin |
| CNTF | Ciliaryneurotrophic Factor |
| IL | Interleukin |
| FGF | Fibroblast Growth Factor |
| GDNF | Glial Cell Line-derived Neurotrophic Factor |
| IGF | Insulin-Like Growth Factor |
| TrkB | Tyrosine Kinase Receptors |
| TNF | Tumor Necrosis Factor |
| TGF-β | Transforming Growth Factor β |
| FFMT | Free Functional Muscle Transfer |
| SAN | Spinal Accessory Nerve |
| MCN | Musculocutaneous Nerve |
| ICNs | Intercostal Nerves |

| | |
|---|---|
| TRN | Triceps Branch of Radial Nerve |
| MPN | Medial Pectoral Nerve |
| ES | Electrical Stimulation |
| OBPP | Obstetric Brachial Plexus Palsy |
| cAMP | Cyclic Adenosine Monophosphate |
| DRG | Dorsal Root Ganglion |
| PKA | Protein Kinase A |
| CREB | Cyclic-AMP Response Binding Protein |

**Author details**

Lin Yang[1*], Yaxuan Li[2], Qianling Zhang[2], Mengnan Jiang[2] and Jia He[2]

1 Department of Human Anatomy, Zhuhai Campus of Zunyi Medical University, Zhuhai, China

2 Zhuhai Campus of Zunyi Medical University, Zhuhai, China

*Address all correspondence to: aiyzwll@aliyun.com

## References

[1] Rich JA, Newell A, Williams T. Traumatic brachial plexus injury rehabilitation using neuromuscular electrical muscle stimulation in a polytrauma patient. BMJ Case Reports. 2019;12(12):e232107. DOI: 10.1136/bcr-2019-232107

[2] Lieberson WT, Holmquest HJ, D. Scott, et al. Functional electrotherapy: stimulation of the peroneal nerve synchronized with the swing phase of the gait of hemiplegic patients. Archives of Physical Medicine and Rehabilitation. 1961;42:101-105. DOI: 10.2307/2656978

[3] Sun B, Zhou ZM, Zhong YJ. Clinical effect of functional electrical stimulation on hemiplegia in stroke patients. Chinese Journal of Practical Nervous Diseases. 2020; 23(12):1095-1099. DOI: CNKI:SUN:HNSJ.0.2020-12-019

[4] Elzinga K, Tyreman N, Ladak A, et al. Brief electrical stimulation improves nerve regeneration after delayed repair in Sprague Dawley rats. Exp Neurol. 2015;269:142-153. DOI: 10.1016/j.expneurol.2015.03.022

[5] Pejkova S, Filipce V, Peev I, et al. Brachial Plexus Injuries - Review of the Anatomy and the Treatment Options. Pril (Makedon Akad Nauk Umet Odd Med Nauki). 2021;42(1):91-103. DOI: 10.2478/prilozi-2021-0008

[6] Hsueh YH, Tu YK. Surgical reconstructions for adult brachial plexus injuries. Part I: Treatments for combined C5 and C6 injuries, with or without C7 injuries. Injury. 2020; 51(4):787-803. DOI: 10.1016/j.injury.2020.02.076

[7] Jang SY, Shin YK, Park SY, et al. Autophagic myelin destruction by Schwann cells during Wallerian degeneration and segmental demyelination. Glia. 2016;64(5):730-742. DOI: 10.1002/glia.22957

[8] Barton MJ, John JS, Clarke M, et al. The Glia Response after Peripheral Nerve Injury: A Comparison between Schwann Cells and Olfactory Ensheathing Cells and Their Uses for Neural Regenerative Therapies. Int J Mol Sci. 2017 Jan 29;18(2):287. DOI: 10.3390/ijms18020287

[9] Chao MV. Neurotrophins and their receptors: a convergence point for many signalling pathways. Nat Rev Neurosci. 2003 Apr;4(4):299-309. DOI: 10.1038/nrn1078

[10] Chen ZY, Chai YF, Cao L, et al. Glial cell line-derived neurotrophic factor enhances axonal regeneration following sciatic nerve transection in adult rats. Brain Res. 2001;902(2):272-276. DOI: 10.1016/s0006-8993(01)02395-2

[11] Omura T, Sano M, Omura K, et al. Different expressions of BDNF, NT3, and NT4 in muscle and nerve after various types of peripheral nerve injuries. J Peripher Nerv Syst. 2005; 10(3):293-300. DOI: 10.1111/j.1085-9489.2005.10307.x

[12] Faustino C, Rijo P, Reis CP. Nanotechnological strategies for nerve growth factor delivery: Therapeutic implications in Alzheimer's disease. Pharmacol Res. 2017 Jun;120:68-87. DOI: 10.1016/j.phrs.2017.03.020

[13] Song KK, Zhang K, Jia L. The microenvironment and repair methods of peripheral nervous system injury. J Clin Rehabil Tis Eng Res. 2021; No.933(04):165-170. DOI: CNKI:SUN:XDKF.0.2021-04-031

[14] Austin PJ, Moalem-Taylor G. The neuro-immune balance in neuropathic pain: Involvement of inflammatory immune cells, immune-like glial cells and cytokines. Journal of Neuroimmunology. 2010;229(1-2):26-50. DOI: 10.1016/j.jneuroim.2010.08.013

[15] Rotshenker S. Wallerian degeneration: the innate-immune response to traumatic nerve injury. Journal of Neuroinflammation. 2011;8(1):1-14. DOI: 10.1186/1742-2094-8-109

[16] Nadeau S, Filali M, Zhang J, et al. Functional recovery after peripheral nerve injury is dependent on the pro-inflammatory cytokines IL-1βand TNF: implications for neuropathic pain. J Neurosci. 2011;31(35):12533-12542. DOI: 10.1523/JNEUROSCI.2840-11.2011

[17] Gaudet AD, Popovich PG, Ramer MS. Wallerian degeneration: gaining perspective on inflammatory events after peripheral nerve injury. J Neuroinflammation. 2011;8:110. DOI: 10.1186/1742-2094-8-110

[18] Yu HJ, Fei J, Chen XS, et al. Progesterone attenuates neurological behavioral deficits of experimental autoimmune encephalomyelitis through remyelination with nucleus-sublocalized Olig1 protein. Neurosci Lett. 2010;476(1):42-45. DOI: 10.1016/j.neulet.2010.03.079

[19] Li WW, Le Goascogne C, Schumacher M, et al. Type 2 deiodinase in the peripheral nervous system: induction in the sciatic nerve after injury. Neuroscience. 2001;107(3):507-518. DOI: 10.1016/s0306-4522(01)00362-1

[20] Mohammadi R, Yadegarazadi MJ, Amini K. Peripheral nerve regeneration following transection injury to rat sciatic nerve by local application of adrenocorticotropic hormone. J Craniomaxillofac Surg. 2014;42(6):784-789. DOI: 10.1016/j.jcms.2013.11.012

[21] Bertelli JA, Ghizoni MF. Combined injury of the accessory nerve and brachial plexus. Neurosurgery. 2011;68(2):390-395; discussion 396. DOI: 10.1227/NEU.0b013e318201d7d9

[22] Xiao C, Lao J, Wang T, et al. Intercostal nerve transfer to neurotize the musculocutaneous nerve after traumatic brachial plexus avulsion: a comparison of two, three, and four nerve transfers. J Reconstr Microsurg. 2014;30(5):297-304. DOI: 10.1055/s-0033-1361840

[23] Songcharoen P, Wongtrakul S, Spinner RJ. Brachial plexus injuries in the adult. nerve transfers: the Siriraj Hospital experience. Hand Clin. 2005;21(1):83-89. DOI: 10.1016/j.hcl.2004.10.002

[24] Gu YD, Zhang GM, Chen DS, et al. Seventh cervical nerve root transfer from the contralateral healthy side for treatment of brachial plexus root avulsion. J Hand Surg Br. 1992;17(5):518-521. DOI: 10.1016/s0266-7681(05)80235-9

[25] Oberlin C, Béal D, Leechavengvongs S, et al. Nerve transfer to biceps muscle using a part of ulnar nerve for C5-C6 avulsion of the brachial plexus: anatomical study and report of four cases. J Hand Surg Am. 1994;19(2):232-237. DOI: 10.1016/0363-5023(94)90011-6

[26] Blaauw G, Slooff AC. Transfer of pectoral nerves to the musculocutaneous nerve in obstetric upper brachial plexus palsy. Neurosurgery. 2003;53(2):338-341. DOI: 10.1227/01.neu.0000073420.66113.66

[27] Ray WZ, Yarbrough CK, Yee A, et al. Clinical outcomes following brachialis to anterior interosseous nerve transfers. J Neurosurg. 2012;117(3):604-609. DOI: 10.3171/2012.6.JNS111332

[28] Maldonado AA, Kircher MF, Spinner RJ, et al. Free Functioning Gracilis Muscle Transfer versus Intercostal Nerve Transfer to Musculocutaneous Nerve for Restoration of Elbow Flexion after

Traumatic Adult Brachial Pan-Plexus Injury. Plast Reconstr Surg. 2016;138(3):483e-488e. DOI: 10.1097/PRS.0000000000002471

[29] Liu SZ, Zhao S, Zhao WY. et al. Effect of early rehabilitation on neonatal brachial plexus injury. J Hebei Med Univ. 2016;37(1):27-29. DOI: 10.3969/j.issn.1007-3205.2016.01.008

[30] Popovic MR, Popovic DB, Keller T. Neuroprostheses for grasping. Neurol Res. 2002 Jul;24(5):443-452. DOI: 10.1179/016164102101200311

[31] Cameron T. Safety and efficacy of spinal cord stimulation for the treatment of chronic pain: a 20-year literature review. J Neurosurg. 2004;100(3 Suppl Spine):254-67. DOI: 10.3171/spi.2004.100.3.0254

[32] Huang J, Lu L, Hu X, et al. Electrical stimulation accelerates motor functional recovery in the rat model of 15-mm sciatic nerve gap bridged by scaffolds with longitudinally oriented microchannels. Neurorehabil Neural Repair. 2010;24(8):736-745. DOI: 10.1177/1545968310368686

[33] Asensio-Pinilla E, Udina E, Jaramillo J, Navarro X. Electrical stimulation combined with exercise increase axonal regeneration after peripheral nerve injury. Exp Neurol. 2009;219(1):258-265. DOI: 10.1016/j.expneurol.2009.05.034

[34] Yeh CC, Lin YC, Tsai FJ, et al. Timing of applying electrical stimulation is an important factor deciding the success rate and maturity of regenerating rat sciatic nerves. Neurorehabil Neural Repair. 2010;24(8):730-735. DOI: 10.1177/1545968310376758

[35] Al-Majed AA, Brushart TM, Gordon T. Electrical stimulation accelerates and increases expression of BDNF and trkB mRNA in regenerating rat femoral motoneurons. Eur J Neurosci. 2000;12(12):4381-4390. DOI: 10.1111/j.1460-9568.2000.01341.x

[36] Al-Majed AA, Tam SL, Gordon T. Electrical stimulation accelerates and enhances expression of regeneration-associated genes in regenerating rat femoral motoneurons. Cell Mol Neurobiol. 2004;24(3):379-402. DOI: 10.1023/b:cemn.0000022770.66463.f7

[37] Zanakis MF. Differential effects of various electrical parameters onperi pheral and central nerve regeneration. Acupunct Electrother Res. 1990;15(3-4):185-191. DOI: info:doi/10.3727/036012990816358199

[38] Shen NJ, Wang SC. Using a direct current electrical field to promotespinal-cord regeneration. J Reconstr Microsurg. 1999;15(6):427-431. DOI: 10.1055/s-2007-1000122

[39] Lu MC, Tsai CC, Chen SC, et al. Use of electrical stimulation at different current levels to promote recovery after peripheral nerve injury in rats. J Trauma. 2009;67(5):1066-1072. DOI: 10.1097/TA.0b013e318182351a

[40] Marquez-Chin C, Popovic MR. Functional electrical stimulation therapy for restoration of motor function after spinal cord injury and stroke: a review. Biomed Eng Online. 2020;19(1):34. DOI: 10.1186/s12938-020-00773-4

[41] Joubert KE. Electrical nerve stimulation as an aid to the placement of a brachial plexus block. J S Afr Vet Assoc. 2002;73(4):216-218. DOI: 10.4102/jsava.v73i4.590

[42] Zhao XJ, Lu SC, Xu P. Application of Nerve Stimulation Instrument Guided Interscalene Brachial Plexus Nerve Block Anesthesia in Upper Limb Surgery. Chin Cont Med Edu. 2017,

009(023):72-73. DOI:10.3969/j.issn.1674-9308.2017.23.037

[43] Shapira Y, Midha R. Shocking therapy: Brief electrical stimulation for delayed nerve repair. Exp Neurol. 2015;271:524-525. DOI: 10.1016/j.expneurol.2015.07.015

[44] Chen YL, Deng M, Li JG, et al. Clinical study of percutaneous positioning of nerve stimulator for intermuscular sulcus brachial plexus block. Chinese Journal of Practical Nervous Diseases. 2016;19(01):82-83. DOI: 10.3969/j.issn.1673-5110.2016.01.045

[45] Liu SZ, Zhao S, Zhao WY, et al. Observation on the effect of early rehabilitation on neonatal brachial plexus injury. Journal of Hebei Medical University. 2016;37(01):27-29. DOI: 10.3969/j.issn.1007-3205.2016.01.008

[46] Liu H. Effect of neuromuscular electrical stimulation combined with acupuncture in rehabilitation treatment of brachial plexus injury in children. Guide of China Medicine. 2017;15(14):104-105. DOI: CNKI:SUN:YYXK.0.2017-14-083

[47] Zhou JM, Gu YD, Xu XJ, et al. Clinical research of comprehensive rehabilitation in treating brachial plexus injury patients. Chinese Medical Journal. 2012;125(14):2516-2520. DOI: 10.3760/cma.j.issn.0366-6999.2012.14.022

[48] Ciaramitaro P, Padua L, Devigili G, et al. Prevalence of Neuropathic Pain in Patients with Traumatic Brachial Plexus Injury: A Multicenter Prospective Hospital-Based Study. Pain Med. 2017;18(12):2428-2432. DOI: 10.1093/pm/pnw360

[49] Sun YL, Lin CX, Zhao XC, et al. .Application of electrical stimulation in the nursing and management of patients with brachial plexus injury and pain. World Latest Medicine Information. 2017;17(A3):170-171. DOI: CNKI:SUN:WMIA.0.2017-A3-116

[50] Zuo KJ, Shafa G, Antonyshyn K, et al. A single session of brief electrical stimulation enhances axon regeneration through nerve autografts. Exp Neurol. 2020;323:113074. DOI: 10.1016/j.expneurol.2019.113074

[51] Cobianchi S, Casals-Diaz L, Jaramillo J, et al. Differential effects of activity dependent treatments on axonal regeneration and neuropathic pain after peripheral nerve injury. Exp Neurol. 2013;240:157-167. DOI: 10.1016/j.expneurol.2012.11.023

[52] Huang J, Zhang Y, Lu L, et al. Electrical stimulation accelerates nerve regeneration and functional recovery in delayed peripheral nerve injury in rats. Eur J Neurosci. 2013;38(12):3691-3701. DOI: 10.1111/ejn.12370

[53] He L, Lv MX, Ruan L, et al. An animal experimental study on low-frequency electrical stimulation to promote peripheral nerve regeneration and functional recovery. J Hebei Med Univ.2019;40(4):396-400,405. DOI:10.3969/j.issn.1007-3205.2019.04.005.

[54] Wenjin W, Wenchao L, Hao Z, et al. Electrical stimulation promotes BDNF expression in spinal cord neurons through Ca(2+)- and Erk-dependent signaling pathways. Cell Mol Neurobiol. 2011;31(3):459-467. DOI: 10.1007/s10571-010-9639-0

[55] Urbanchek MG, Kung TA, Frost CM, et al. Development of a Regenerative Peripheral Nerve Interface for Control of a Neuroprosthetic Limb. Biomed Res Int. 2016;2016:5726730. DOI: 10.1155/2016/5726730

[56] Aglah C, Gordon T, Posse de Chaves EI. cAMP promotes neurite outgrowth and extension through

protein kinase A but independently of Erk activation in cultured rat motoneurons. Neuropharmacology. 2008;55(1):8-17. DOI: 10.1016/j.neuropharm.2008.04.005

[57] Batty NJ, Fenrich KK, Fouad K. The role of cAMP and its downstream targets in neurite growth in the adult nervous system. Neurosci Lett. 2017;652:56-63. DOI: 10.1016/j.neulet.2016.12.033

[58] Nakagawa K, Tamaki H, Hayao K, et al. Electrical Stimulation of Denervated Rat Skeletal Muscle Retards Capillary and Muscle Loss in Early Stages of Disuse Atrophy. Biomed Res Int. 2017;2017:5695217. DOI: 10.1155/2017/5695217

[59] Willand MP, Holmes M, Bain JR, et al. Electrical muscle stimulation after immediate nerve repair reduces muscle atrophy without affecting reinnervation. Muscle Nerve. 2013;48(2):219-225. DOI: 10.1002/mus.23726

[60] Zhuang Y, Sun KX, Zhou JM, et al. Clinical observation on the treatment of brachial plexus injury by electroacupuncture combined with rehabilitation training. Chinese Journal of Rehabilitation. 2016;31(2):149-150. DOI: 10.3870/zgkf.2016.02.022

[61] Williams HB. A clinical pilot study to assess functional return following continuous muscle stimulation after nerve injury and repair in the upper extremity using a completely implantable electrical system. Microsurgery. 1996;17(11):597-605. DOI: 10.1002/(SICI)1098-2752(1996)17:113.0.CO;2-M

[62] Gordon T. Electrical Stimulation to Enhance Axon Regeneration After Peripheral Nerve Injuries in Animal Models and Humans. Neuro therapeutics. 2016;13(2):295-310. DOI: 10.1007/s13311-015-0415-1

[63] Menorca RM, Fussell TS, Elfar JC. Nerve physiology: mechanisms of injury and recovery. Hand Clin. 2013; 29(3):317-330. DOI: 10.1016/j.hcl.2013.04.002

[64] Paillard, and Thierry. "Muscle plasticity of aged subjects in response to electrical stimulation training and inversion and/or limitation of the sarcopenic process." Ageing Research Reviews (2018):S1568163718300667.

[65] Honda Y, Tanaka N, Kajiwara Y, et al. Effect of belt electrode-skeletal muscle electrical stimulation on immobilization-induced muscle fibrosis. PLoS One. 2021;16(5):e0244120. DOI: 10.1371/journal.pone.0244120

Section 4

# Outcome

Chapter 6

# Outcome Measures in OBPP

*Shivani Gupta, Nivetha Srinivasan, Jasmine Mahajan, Amy Song, Alice Chu and Aleksandra McGrath*

## Abstract

Traditional outcome measurement scales, such as the Medical Research Council (MRC) score, the Active Movement Scale (AMS), and Mallet score, are used by surgeons to assess outcomes in patients with obstetric brachial plexus palsy (OBPP). The measurement scales used to evaluate patients fall under the International Classification of Functioning (ICF) domains of Body Function, Body Structure, Activity, Participation, and Environment and are used to assess function and disability of patients. Currently used outcome measures scales for OBPP are also contrasted with those used for another perinatal condition affecting the upper limb, cerebral palsy (CP).

**Keywords:** brachial plexus injury, brachial plexus palsy, evaluation measurement, international classification, outcome assessment

## 1. Introduction

Patients with OBPP are treated with a multidisciplinary approach. As soon as the diagnosis is suspected, patients are referred to neurology, as well as physical and occupational therapy. Rehabilitation focuses on contracture prevention, including passive range of motion exercises at relevant joints, supportive splints for elbows and hand, and muscle strengthening exercises to promote normal function [1, 2]. Primary or secondary surgical intervention is indicated in cases of severe nerve injury and absent or suboptimal functional recovery. Interventions include nerve microsurgery, joint and bony procedures, tendon lengthening and transfers [3]. Post-operative management after nerve surgery can also include electrical muscle stimulation to facilitate muscle function [4]. Botulinum toxin injections can be used to treat muscle imbalance and contractures. A systematic review identified 4 groups of indicators for botulinum injection: contracture of shoulder adduction, limited active elbow flexion and extension, and pronation contracture of the lower arm [5]. However, specific indications for nerve repair or secondary surgery are largely institution-specific due to a lack of randomized trials and multicenter prospective studies.

Outcomes are often difficult to compare due to the variability of anatomical lesions, variety in surgical technique, and difference in outcome reporting [6]. While the majority of OBPP outcome measurements focus on the functional limitation of the upper extremity, affected children often have associated psychosocial problems, most commonly in the area of activity and participation, such as sports [7]. In comparison to healthy children, children with OBPP have been found to be at high risk for anxiety, depression, and aggression. Mothers with children with OBPP

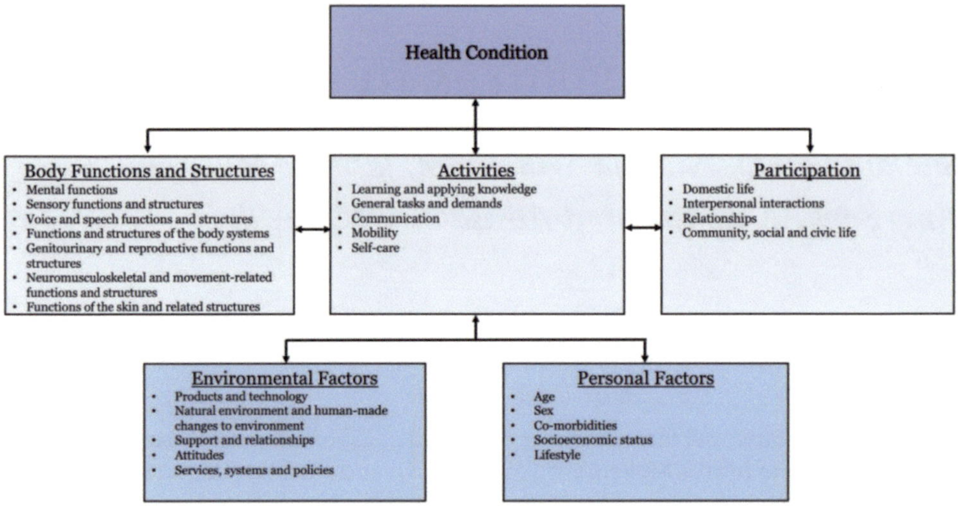


**Figure 1.**
*Integrated ICF Model [9].*

have been found to have increased maternal distress compared to mothers with healthy children [8].

The International Classification of Functioning, Disability and Health (ICF) is a validated and valuable tool developed by the World Health Organization for identifying and comparing areas of function and disability of persons in several domains. The ICF framework consists of five domains: body structure, body function, activity, participation, and environmental factors [9]. These domains are detailed in the integrated biopsychosocial model in **Figure 1**. The activity domain evaluates task execution in the context of disablement or physical ability. The participation domain addresses patient involvement in activities of daily living (ADL) or patient self-perception of engagement and psychometric well-being [10]. Children, adolescents, and young adults with OBPP are important stakeholders, and the application of holistic OBPP evaluation that measures various ICF domains can help improve understanding of their situation. In this chapter, we describe all currently used outcome measures for OBPP, map them against domains in International Classification of Functioning, Disability and Health, and contrast OBPP with another perinatal condition affecting the upper limb, cerebral palsy (CP).

## 2. Outcomes in OBPP

### 2.1 Traditional OBPP outcome measures

With the onset of World War I and II alongside the spread of poliomyelitis, surgeons and neurologists saw a rapid increase in peripheral nerve injuries in the hospitals. A majority of these cases affected the upper limb, including brachial plexus lesions. In response, the British Medical Research Council (MRC) created the MRC score to examine the limbs for peripheral nerve lesions as seen in **Table 1**. It tested limb segment positioning without and against gravity, and manual resistance was tested to grade muscle strength on a six point scale measuring no activity, flicker, movement with gravity eliminated, movement against gravity, and normal power. Grade 4 is subdivided into 3 categories: slight, moderate, and strong resistance. However, these subdivisions are subjective and thus, levels of resistance are highly

| **MRC score** | |
|---|---|
| **Grade** | **Clinical Finding** |
| 0 | No contraction |
| 1 | Flicker, trace of contraction |
| 2 | Active movement with gravity eliminated |
| 3 | Active movement against gravity |
| 4 | Active movement against gravity and resistance |
| 5 | Normal power |

**Table 1.**
*MRC score [11].*

dependent on the evaluator [11]. The MRC scale has become the most recognized scale for evaluating strength in patients with peripheral nerve injuries, and it is commonly used for assessing elbow flexion in infants with OBPP [12–16]. Individual surgeons often develop and use their own modifications for documenting results, especially for how grade 4 can be defined for different movements or muscles.

Over time, the Gilbert Muscle Grading System emerged in 1987 to address MRC's limitations with manual resistance as seen in **Table 2**. It evaluates shoulder function on a 0–5 point scale, representing: flaccid, no active external rotation (ER) at abduction to 45°, no active ER at abduction to <90°, weak active ER at abduction to 90°, weak active ER at abduction to <120°, and complete active ER at abduction to >120° [17]. The Gilbert shoulder abduction sub score can be converted into the Mallet shoulder abduction sub score by utilizing the corresponding range of motion [18]. In both cases, the MRC scale is not suitable for infants due to the cognitive requirement for the exam [19].

The Miami scale was developed to address the limitation in choosing a grade within the Gilbert system. It totals the score for shoulder abduction and external rotation to calculate a grade of 0–5, where 0 represents no function and 5 is excellent. This score has been found to have a weak correlation with Gilbert and Mallet, but it has not been validated for OBPP [20].

A decade earlier, the Mallet score was created in 1972 to evaluate OBPP injuries on a scale of 1–5 by testing functionality of the affected limb as seen in **Table 3** [21]. Commonly used to assess shoulder abduction before and after surgery, the Mallet score translates grade of shoulder external rotation into degrees of deficiency. A score of 1 corresponds to a flail shoulder and a score of 5 indicating a normal shoulder [22]. The Mallet classification system includes 5 sub scores for shoulder movements: abduction, external rotation, hand to neck, hand on spine, and hand to mouth, to give a maximum score of 25. Active range of motion measurements can be translated into the Mallet scale [21].

Modified versions of the Mallet scale have also been created. In addition to the classical shoulder assessments of the Mallet system, Birch's modified Mallet system evaluates resting position and fixed forearm supination on a scale of 1–5, with 1 being most affected and 5 being normal [23]. Nath et al's modified Mallet system integrates Birch's modification to further define deformity [24]. Terzis and Papakonstantinou created a modified Mallet scale that measures the same shoulder movements as the original Mallet scale, but it uses a scale of 1–4 [25]. Abzug et al's modification measures a 6th sub score to the original Mallet system: hand to belly; this additional internal rotation position improves assessment of postoperative midline function [26, 27].

| Gilbert Shoulder Classification | |
|---|---|
| **Grade (Function)** | **Clinical Finding** |
| 0 (none) | Flaccid shoulder |
| 1 (poor) | No active external rotation at abduction to 45° |
| 2 (fair) | No external rotation at abduction to 90° |
| 3 (satisfactory) | Weak active external rotation at abduction to 90° |
| 4 (good) | Weak active external rotation at abduction to <120° |
| 5 (excellent) | Complete active external rotation at abduction to >120° |

**Table 2.**
*Gilbert Shoulder Classification [17].*

| Mallet Score | |
|---|---|
| **Grade** | **Clinical Finding** |
| I | Flail shoulder |
| II | 0° of external rotation<br>Active abduction <30°<br>Hand to mouth with marked trumpet sign<br>Hand to back of neck impossible<br>Hand to back impossible |
| III | External rotation < 20°<br>Active abduction 30°– 90°<br>Hand to mouth possible with partial trumpet sign (> 40° shoulder abduction)<br>Hand to back of neck with difficulty<br>Hand to back with difficulty |
| IV | External rotation > 20°<br>Active abduction > 90°<br>Hand to mouth easy with <40° shoulder abduction<br>Hand to back of neck easy<br>Hand to back easy |
| V | Normal shoulder |

**Table 3.**
*Mallet score [21].*

After noting the deficiencies in the Mallet and MRC scoring systems, the active movement scale (AMS) was created in 1995 as a novel evaluative tool to be used on infants and children at any time point (**Table 4**). While a child is playing, upper limb movement is observed in the gravity-eliminated and anti-gravity planes. At the shoulder, abduction, and adduction, flexion, external rotation, internal rotation are tested; at the elbow, flexion and extension; at the forearm, pronation and supination; at the wrist, finger, and thumb, flexion and extension. AMS is quantified on an 8 point scale (0 for no visible contraction to 7 for full motion) based on the percent of active motion noted within individual joint passive range of motion [28]. It is recommended that the estimated passive range of motion (PROM) be verified with goniometry for accurate scoring [29]. It has showed moderate to excellent reliability in children with OBPP between 1 month and 15 years of age [30]. Active range of motion measurements can be reliably converted to the AMS scale. The extended numerical scale improves distinguishing ability and allows for extended statistical analysis.

However, upper-extremity movements of forearm pronation and supination are less reliably evaluated with AMS [19]. AMS has been shown to be more popular in North America while Europe has shown preference towards MRC. Although it has been shown to work on an extended age range, AMS is typically used in younger children [31]. Though this is the case, AMS is often time consuming in younger children as it requires patience and creativity from the provider and cooperation from the child to elicit all the desired motions [32].

The Toronto Test Score was created in 1994 to predict a child's prognosis prior to microsurgical intervention (**Table 5**). Shoulder flexion, extension, abduction, and external rotation is measured; elbow flexion, radioulnar supination, and wrist extension is also recorded. On a scale of 0 (no motion or contraction) to 7 (full motion), if a 3 month child scores < 3.5, this result recommends nerve surgery [33]. It has been validated for use in children with OBPP. Composite Toronto and AMS scores have demonstrated a strong correlation [34].

In 1993, the Raimondi hand and wrist score was developed specifically for OBPP with a scale ranging from 1, for total palsy, to 5, for nearly normal hand function (**Table 6**). By incorporating sensation and motor function in its evaluation, the Raimondi scale is able to determine extent of hand function [35]. The Gilbert-Raimondi score classifies elbow function in OBPP by analyzing flexion, extension,

| **AMS Score** | |
|---|---|
| **Grade** | **Clinical Finding** |
| 0 | Gravity eliminated: no contraction |
| 1 | Gravity eliminated: contraction, no motion |
| 2 | Gravity eliminated: motion < ½ range |
| 3 | Gravity eliminated: Motion > ½ range |
| 4 | Gravity eliminated: full motion |
| 5 | Against gravity: motion < ½ range |
| 6 | Against gravity: motion > ½ range |
| 7 | Against gravity: full motion |

**Table 4.**
*AMS Score [28].*

| **Toronto Score** | | |
|---|---|---|
| **Grade** | **Clinical Finding** | **Score** |
| 0 | Gravity eliminated: no contraction | 0 |
| 1 | Gravity eliminated: contraction, no motion | .3 |
| 2 | Gravity eliminated: motion < ½ range | .3 |
| 3 | Gravity eliminated: Motion > ½ range | .6 |
| 4 | Gravity eliminated: full motion | .6 |
| 5 | Against gravity: motion < ½ range | .6 |
| 6 | Against gravity: motion > ½ range | 1.3 |
| 7 | Against gravity: full motion | 2 |

**Table 5.**
*Toronto Test Score [33].*

| Raimondi Hand Score | |
|---|---|
| **Grade** | **Clinical Finding** |
| 0 | Complete paralysis or functionally useless finger flexion<br>Non-usable thumbs without grasping function<br>Little or no sensation |
| 1 | Limited finger flexion<br>No finger or wrist extension<br>Key grip possible |
| 2 | Active wrist extension<br>Passive flexion of fingers (tenodesis)<br>Passive key grip in pronation |
| 3 | Complete active finger and wrist flexion<br>Active thumb movement, including abduction and opposition<br>Intrinsic equilibrium<br>No active supination |
| 4 | Complete active finger and wrist flexion<br>Active wrist extension but weak finger extension<br>Good opposition of thumb with active ulnar intrinsic muscles<br>Partial pronation and supination |
| 5 | Grade 4, but with active finger extension<br>Complete pronation and supination |

**Table 6.**
*Raimondi Hand Score [35].*

and lack of extension to assign a value of I (poor recovery), II (satisfactory recovery) or III (good recovery) [36]. Gilbert-Raimondi can also be used to classify hand function on a scale of 0 to 5 [37].

Active range of motion (AROM) has shown to have the largest support from the international brachial plexus surgeon community according to the iPLUTO study [31]. It has a continuous scale and normative values are readily available. However, the methodology in assessment varies. Some use goniometers for a precise measurement; however, it is cumbersome to use, especially with a fussy child. Passive range of motion (PROM) is also commonly assessed and reported as these children commonly develop internal rotation shoulder and elbow flexion contractures [31].

Traditional surgeon- or therapist-reported physical exam outcome measures, like Mallet, Toronto, and AMS, have been validated for OBPP and can discriminate the deficit in active range of motion in the upper extremity [30]. However, these scales focus primarily on individual muscle power. Systematic review has shown that measures of shoulder or elbow range of motion are most frequently used for outcome assessment for OBPP [38]. Notably, a study surveyed attendees of the International Symposium of Brachial Plexus Surgery over the course of nine months. Fifty-nine participants responded and all but two were surgeons. Most responders were based in Europe or North America and identified as a member of a brachial plexus team. There was a consensus (76%) to include passive range of motion for shoulder adduction and abduction and elbow extension. 95% of respondents believed active range motion should also be measured by evaluating shoulder abduction and adduction, elbow flexion and extension, wrist extension, and finger flexion and extension. 83% expressed that the Mallet score was a suitable outcome measure, and 76% said it should be expressed using its sub scores for each movement, rather than using an aggregate score. There was also insufficient evidence for the use of Azbug et al's modified Mallet scale, which includes hand-to-belly to assess active internal rotation [31].

### 2.2 Importance of ICF framework

At each age group, there is a different motivation for assessment. During infancy, the degree of impairment is identified and recovery is monitored to determine qualification for surgery; thus, range of motion, strength, and limb integration must be evaluated. As the child develops, the assessment must evolve with them. For a school-aged patient, participation in age-related school and leisure activities as well as qualify of life is important to their development. Adolescents with OBPP may face functional limitations stemming from factors that these surgeon-centered outcome measures do not assess, such as psychosocial factors, poor self-perception, or social environmental influences [39]. While functional impairment must also be measured, psychometric assessment must now be included to holistically measure OBPP outcomes [10].

Several tools have been developed for global clinical assessment that evaluate domains aside from "body function and structure", which has been well documented by the MRC, Mallet, and AMS scales. The Brachial Plexus Outcome Measure (BPOM) activity scale, specific for school-aged children with OBPP, measures function relative to activity limitations stemming from brachial plexus nerve injury. It consists of eleven tasks, which contain components of the fifteen movements used in the AMS scale, and performance is graded using the Functional Movement Scale ranging from 1 to 5. Patients fill out the self-evaluation scale with 3 visual analog scales to score perceived hand and arm function as well as aesthetic appearance of the affected limb [40]. BPOM measures a component of the ICF definition of participation by considering the child's upper limb performance within the context of their life [38]. Its authors recommend clinicians to supplement the BPOM activity scale with a global standardized participation questionnaire when needed to measure the ICF "activity and participation" domain [40].

Sensory discriminatory function in patients with OBPP can be evaluated using Semmes-Weinstein monofilaments and two-point discrimination. The Semmes-Weinstein monofilament test uses five monofilaments of different diameters, where thicker filaments exert higher pressure when applied to skin [41]. Behavior cues, such as retractive movements with active motion and facial grimacing, in response to pinprick across dermatomes can be classified using the Sensory Grading Scale by Narakas when testing infants [10]. It is classified under the "body function" ICF domain [38].

Noting the lack of sensitivity of the Gilbert-Raimondi hand classification, the nine hole peg test has been validated to evaluate fine upper motor function in patients with OBPP [42]. It requires participants to repeatedly place and subsequently remove nine pegs into nine holes one at a time, as fast as they can. This test has shown to have high interrater and test–retest reliability for both the adult and pediatric population [43]. It is classified under the "activity" ICF domain [44]. However, the iPLUTO survey showed a consensus to not use this tool [31]. Recognizing the dynamics of a dominant and assisting hand in bimanual hand activity, the Assisting Hand Assessment (AHA) was developed in 2003 as a hand function evaluation tool for children with unilateral upper limb dysfunction, including those with OBPP and cerebral palsy (CP). It has been shown to be reliable in children between ages of 18 months and 12 years. Classified under the "activity" ICF domain, the AHA reflects the person's usual performance in daily activities [45].

The Children's Hand-use Experience Questionnaire (CHEQ), a tool for evaluating hand function in unilateral upper limb injury, covers the level of activity in the ICF framework. It is administered in two steps. First, a play session requiring bimanual handling of 22 specific toys is observed; then, the session is reviewed by trained assessors to rate each object-related action on a 4-point scale. It is unique as the questionnaire includes the child's emotional experience of impaired hand function in bimanual activities. Validity has been demonstrated in adolescents aged 6–18 years with OBPP and CP. It should be noted that ratings for children under 13 years of age are completed by parents, who tend to overestimate their child's problems [46].

Disability is commonly assessed by the Disabilities of the Arm, Shoulder, and Hand (DASH) outcome measure in brachial plexus injuries. It is a 30 item, self-reported questionnaire measuring physical function where every question is answered on a scale from 1 to 5, and the total minimum score ranges between 30 and 150 [47]. It has shown responsiveness and validity across the whole upper extremity in adults and covers the "activity and participation" ICF domain [48, 49]. A shorter version, QuickDASH, is comprised of 11 items assessed on a 5-point scale; it has shown higher discriminatory power in detecting disability and has been proven as a valid instrument for children ages 8–18 [50].

To determine arm and hand spontaneous function in the home environment, the parent-reported Hand Use at Home (HUH) questionnaire was developed, which is categorized under the activity and participation of ICF. It includes a host of bimanual activities and has been validated in children aged 3–10 years with unilateral cerebral palsy and OBPP [51].

The Pediatric Outcomes Data Collection Instrument (PODCI) was developed to provide a standardized outcome measurement for pediatric musculoskeletal conditions, and it has been validated for OBPP [52]. The tool has seven dimensions: upper extremity function, transfers and mobility, physical function and sports, comfort or lack of pain, happiness, satisfaction, and expectations [53]. It falls under the "activity, participation, and environmental" domains of the ICF framework [38].

The 36 item Pediatric Quality of Life Inventory, PedsQL, assesses the impact of a child's chronic condition on the family, where a higher score represents low impact [54]. It is developed for pediatric patients with chronic health conditions. It is a promising health-related quality of life instrument designed for a broad age range, including categories for both parents and patients. It measures the core health dimensions outlined by the WHO, including functionality at school [55]. This measurement is a validated outcome measure that is categorized under the "activity and participation" ICF domain [44].

Patient-Reported Outcomes Measurement Information System (PROMIS) developed by the NIH includes several measures to holistically evaluate physical, mental, and social health [56]. The health quality of children with obstetric brachial plexus palsy as measured by PROMIS is not well understood. For other brachial plexus related injuries, such as brachial plexus birth injury, PROMIS domains have shown promise as useful tools for evaluation [56].

A summary of OBPP outcome measure classification by ICF domain can be found in **Figure 2**. In a systematic review of classifying OBPP outcome measures by ICF domain, only 8% (18/217) of papers represented the ICF component of "activity and participation" and only 4% (9/217) of studies incorporated the concept of environmental factors during OBPP measurement; the remaining 88% (190/217) studied the ICF domain of "body structure and function". In total, only 2% (4/217) of papers evaluated all three ICF domains [38]. It should be noted that the ICF framework does not include the impact of the child's disability on the family. Family members have been found to experience "third-party functioning and disability" as a result of their loved one's health condition [57].

### 2.3 OBPP evaluation contrasted with CP evaluation

Similar to OBPP, children with the most common type of hemiplegic cerebral palsy (HCP) have a weak upper limb from their pre- or perinatal period. In CP, damage or abnormalities of the cerebral motor cortex affects muscle coordination

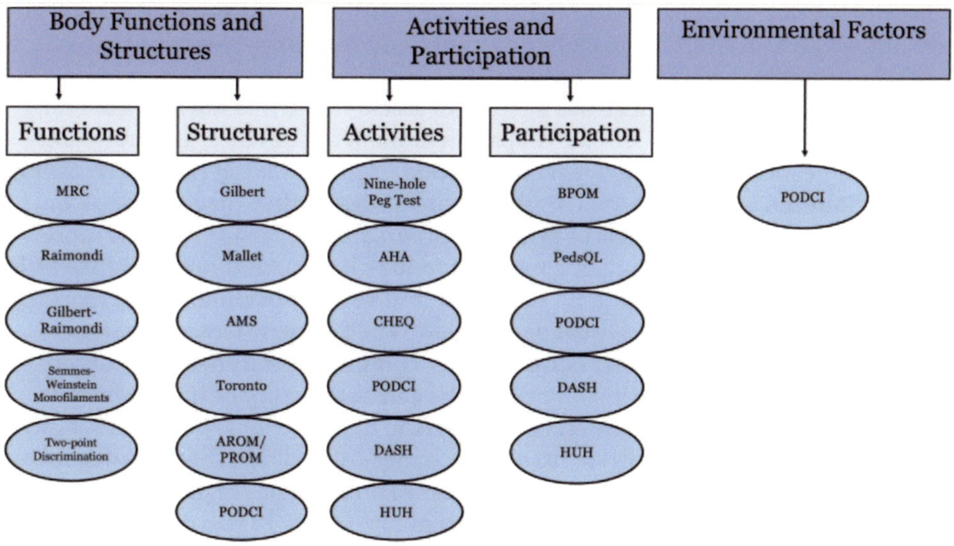


**Figure 2.**
*Classification of OBPP outcome measures by ICF domain.*

and movement. Other central nervous system deficits in HCP include sensory impairments, failure of sensorimotor integration, and potential learning disabilities [58]. There has been extensive study of upper extremity dysfunction in children with CP, including the age at which children plateau in function and the use of multimodal therapeutics such as synergistic Botox, occupational therapy, and augmented feedback therapeutics such as virtual reality [58].

Children with HCP often take longer to complete bimanual activities. They may ask for assistance if they are comfortable or they may avoid certain activities due to negative effects on their self-esteem and self-concept. This interplay between body structure and function with environmental and personal factors again proves the importance of the ICF framework.

Since cerebral palsy and obstetric brachial plexus palsy both exhibit unilateral upper limb palsy, they share several outcome measurements. AROM and PROM are also often measured by goniometry for CP patients, similar to OBPP patients. For both diagnoses, it is important to note that this outcome can be affected by age, gender, baseline level of physical activity, and any co-existing illness. MRC has been utilized for measuring muscle power in CP patients although this was developed initially for brachial plexus lesions [59]. Mean time to complete nine-hole pegboard, which measures finger dexterity, has been used in CP patients as well [60, 61].

Other scales more specific to CP that fall under the "body function and structure" domain of the ICF framework include the Ashworth and Modified Ashworth scales for spasticity and Kendall scale for muscle strength [62]. The Quality of Upper Extremity Skills Test (QUEST) is used to assess the body structure and function domain by taking into consideration disassociated movement, grasp, protective extension, and weight bearing. The test–retest reliability ranges from 0.75 to 0.95 depending on the factor considered [63]. The Melbourne Assessment of Unilateral Upper Limb Function (MUUL) is a video-based measurement with 16 items, each containing subskills that cover various characteristics of movement including target accuracy, fluency, and movement. A score out of 122 is calculated and then converted into a percentage that describes the quality of upper limb movement in CP patients [64]. The Box and Blocks timed test measures unilateral dexterity by having children move blocks from one side a box to another using the dominant hand and the non-dominant hand [65]. The Barry-Albright Dystonia (BAD) scale rates the severity of dystonia in eight different body regions—eyes, mouth, neck, trunk, both arms, and both legs [66].

There are also a variety of scales utilized to assess OBPP that are also used for CP that address the activity and participation domain of the ICF framework. One such outcome measure, as previously mentioned, is the Assisting Hand Assessment (AHA). Children with unilateral CP are videorecorded as they play with toys and/or boardgames that provoke use of both hands and are then assigned a raw score between 22 and 88 which are then converted to logit based AHA units [45]. AHA is often used in research and has good reliability and validity in children but requires extensive training to administer the assessment. The Pediatric Outcomes Data Collection Instrument (PODCI) helps families communicate information about their environment and share how it affects the gait and quality of life of children with musculoskeletal health issues. In comparison to its use for OBPP, PODCI only demonstrates moderate sensitivity to detect changes of walking function due to its expansive scoring system [67]. This outcome measure also has high ceiling effects [68]. Children's Hand-use Experience Questionnaire (CHEQ) was developed to be a useful tool to assess patients who have limitations in one hand making it difficult to perform bimanual activities.

There are other outcome measures that fall under the activity and participation domain used for CP but not OBPP. Pediatric Quality of Life Inventory (PedsQL), a part of the participation ICF domain, is used by families to score their children with CP taking into consideration a variety of other factors that affect life [69–71]. One that falls under the ICF framework is Pediatric Evaluation of Disability Inventory (PEDI). PEDI is administered to children less than seven years of age and is formatted as a semi-structured interview administered by proxy [72]. It assesses for ability to provide self-care and maintain social function. The Canadian Occupational Performance Measure (COPM) is a 5-step process used by occupational therapists to evaluate the effect of therapy on various individualized outcomes of importance such as self-care, productivity, and leisure and rate performance and satisfaction on a scale of 1–10 [73]. Jebsen Taylor Hand Function Test (JTHFT) is a timed test of hand dexterity in everyday activities used in children greater than 5 years of age [74]. Although COPM and JTHFT are not diagnosis specific to CP, they have been utilized to evaluate CP patients over time [74, 75]. PROMIS has also been utilized for CP patient evaluation [76]. The Hand Assessment for Infants (HAI) is used to describe unilateral hand function in CP patients by quantifying the contribution of each hand separately and together during a 10–15-minute play session with specific toys eliciting a wide range of motor actions [77]. Both Hands Assessment (BoHA) is a video-taped tool that was developed for children under 12 years of age with bilateral CP and measures the effectiveness of each individual hand during multiple bimanual tasks. Although the scale is highly precise and captures the mobility subdomain of the activity domain of the ICF framework, it requires administrators to undergo formal training and scoring can be time-intensive [78]. ABILHAND-Kids, from the self-care subdomain of the activity domain, is a questionnaire administered to the parents of CP children, thus leading to possible over- or under-estimation of their child's bimanual everyday activities [78]. The Gross Motor Function Scale (GMFS) evaluates a child's ability to complete basic motor functions such as crawling, jumping, or climbing up stairs on a four point scale for each task [79]. Peabody Developmental Motor Scales second edition (PDMS-2) assesses fine motor skills in children with results expressed as raw scores, standard scores and total motor quotient [80]. Children's Assessment of Participation and Assessment (CAPE) is a 55-item questionnaire administered to the child and parent

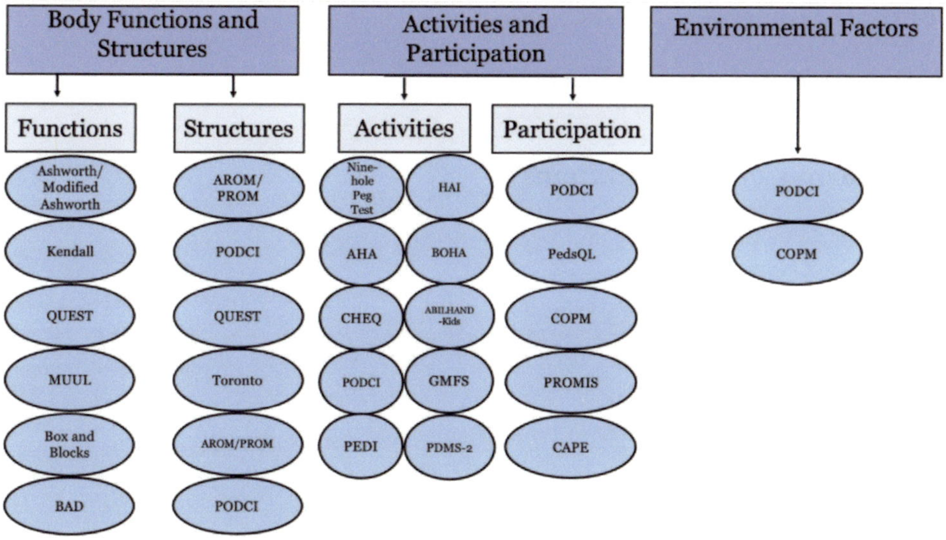


**Figure 3.**
*Classification of CP outcome measures by ICF domain.*

and is designed to examine how children with physical disabilities like CP participate in everyday activities outside of the school setting and document the diversity, intensity, and enjoyment of activities [81].

A summary of CP outcome measure classification by ICF domain can be found in **Figure 3**. There is a discordance between outcome measures that focus on ICF levels of activity and participation and functional measures that attempt to quantify motion. Both OBPP and CP have effects on patients beyond movement and strength. Quality of life, stress to caregivers, involvement in school and family activities, self-image and self-esteem can all be affected, indicating the need for more biopsychosocial approaches. Although capturing outcomes incorporating multiple domains of the ICF framework is beneficial, the amount of time and training required for measures of activity and participation often leads to these outcomes not being utilized to its full extent in the clinical setting. The existing body of literature shows that compared to OBPP surgeons, CP surgeons report on more domains of the ICF framework. Mallet, MRC, AMS, AROM, PROM, and Gilbert are mostly used in reporting outcomes on OBPP patients, putting emphasis on quantifying motion. In CP, more emphasis may be placed on activity and participation due to the added complexity of the diagnosis with neurological involvement.

## 3. Conclusions

Currently, most tools used to assess OBPP progression measure range of motion and strength, which are classified under the body function and structure domain of the ICF model. Numerous instruments have been developed, such as the DASH and PODCI score, to include other factors of disability, like self-perception and functional impairment. However, these scales are not typically included during standard OBPP assessments, in contrast to CP outcome reporting, which generally focuses more on the activity and participation domain of the ICF model. Further standardization and incorporation of outcomes that fall under the activity and participation domain would be beneficial to assess OBPP more holistically.

## Conflict of interest

The authors declare no conflict of interest.

## Notes/thanks/other declarations

None.


## Author details

Shivani Gupta[1], Nivetha Srinivasan[1], Jasmine Mahajan[1], Amy Song[1], Alice Chu[1] and Aleksandra McGrath[2,3]*

1 Department of Orthopedic Surgery, Rutgers-New Jersey Medical School, Newark, NJ, USA

2 Department of Clinical Sciences, Umeå University, Umeå, Sweden

3 Department of Surgical and Perioperative Sciences, Faculty of Medicine, Umeå University, Umeå, Sweden

*Address all correspondence to: aleksandra.mcgrath@umu.se

## References

[1] Volpe JJ. Injuries of Extracranial, Cranial, Intracranial, Spinal Cord, and Peripheral Nervous System Structures. Neurology of the Newborn. 2008;: 959-85.

[2] Yang LJ-S. Neonatal brachial plexus palsy—Management and prognostic factors. Seminars in Perinatology. 2014;38(4):222-34.

[3] Spinner RJ, Kline DG. Surgery for peripheral nerve and brachial plexus injuries or other nerve lesions. Muscle & Nerve. 2000;23(5):680-95.

[4] Chuang DC-C, Ma H-S. Current Concepts in the Management of Obstetrical Brachial Plexus Injuries: The Taipei Experience. Seminars in Plastic Surgery. 2004;18(04):309-17.

[5] Gobets D, Beckerman H, de Groot V, Van Doorn-Loogman MH, Becher JG.Indications and effects of botulinum toxin A for obstetric brachial plexus injury: a systematic literature review. Developmental Medicine & Child Neurology. 2010;52(6):517-28.

[6] T Neonatal brachial plexus palsy. Washington, DC: The American College of Obstetricians and Gynecologists, Women's Health Care Physicians; 2014.

[7] Sarac C, Bastiaansen E, Van der Holst M, Malessy MJ, Nelissen RG, Vliet Vlieland TP. Concepts of functioning and health important to children with an obstetric brachial plexus injury: a qualitative study using focus groups. Developmental Medicine & Child Neurology. 2013;55(12):1136-42.

[8] Alyanak B, Kılınçaslan A, Kutlu L, Bozkurt H, Aydın A. Psychological Adjustment, Maternal Distress, and Family Functioning in Children With Obstetrical Brachial Plexus Palsy. The Journal of Hand Surgery. 2013;38(1): 137-42.

[9] International Classification of Functioning, Disability and Health (ICF) [Internet]. World Health Organization. World Health Organization; [cited 2021Jun1]. Available from: https://www.who.int/standards/classifications/international-classification-of-functioning-disability-and-health

[10] Duff SV, DeMatteo C. Clinical assessment of the infant and child following perinatal brachial plexus injury. Journal of Hand Therapy. 2015;28(2):126-34.

[11] Medical Research Council: Nerve Injuries Committee. Aids to the investigation of peripheral nerve injuries. His Majesty's Stationary Office, London.1942;48

[12] Ghanghurde BA, Mehta R, Ladkat KM, Raut BB, Thatte MR. Distal transfers as a primary treatment in obstetric brachial plexus palsy: a series of 20 cases. Journal of Hand Surgery (European Volume). 2016;41(8):875-81.

[13] Chuang DC-C, Mardini S, Ma H-S. Surgical Strategy for Infant Obstetrical Brachial Plexus Palsy: Experiences at Chang Gung Memorial Hospital. Plastic and Reconstructive Surgery. 2005;116(1):132-42.

[14] Noaman HH, Shiha AE, Bahm J. Oberlin's ulnar nerve transfer to the biceps motor nerve in obstetric brachial plexus palsy: Indications, and good and bad results. Microsurgery. 2004;24(3): 182-7.

[15] Xu J, Cheng X, Gu Y. Different Methods and Results in the Treatment of Obstetrical Brachial Plexus Palsy. Journal of Reconstructive Microsurgery. 2000;16(06):417-22.

[16] Malessy MJA, Pondaag W. Neonatal Brachial Plexus Palsy with Neurotmesis

of C5 and Avulsion of C6. Journal of Bone and Joint Surgery. 2014;96(20).

[17] Terzis JK, Gilbert A, Tassin J-L. In: Microreconstruction of nerve injuries. Philadelphia: Saunders; 1987. p. 529.

[18] Bauer AS, Kalish LA, Adamczyk MJ, Bae DS, Cornwall R, James MA, et al. Microsurgery for Brachial Plexus Injury Before Versus After 6 Months of Age. Journal of Bone and Joint Surgery. 2019;102(3):194-204.

[19] Curtis C, Stephens D, Clarke HM, Andrews D. The active movement scale: An evaluative tool for infants with obstetrical brachial plexus palsy. The Journal of Hand Surgery. 2002;27(3): 470-1.

[20] Grossman JA, DiTaranto P, Price AE, Ramos LE, Tidwell M, Papazian O, et al. Multidisciplinary Management of Brachial Plexus Birth Injuries: The Miami Experience. Seminars in Plastic Surgery. 2004;18(04):319-26.

[21] Mallet J. Obstetrical paralysis of the brachial plexus. II. Therapeutics. Treatment of sequelae. Priority for the treatment of the shoulder. Method for the expression of results. Rev Chir Orthop Reparatrice Appar Mot. 1972;58:166-8.

[22] Al-Qattan MM, El-Sayed AA. Obstetric Brachial Plexus Palsy: The Mallet Grading System for Shoulder Function—Revisited. BioMed Research International. 2014;2014:1-3.

[23] Birch R. Late sequelae at the shoulder in obstetrical palsy in children. In: Randelli M, Karlsson J, editor. Surgical Techniques in Orthopaedics and Traumatology: Shoulder. Vol. 3. Paris: Elsevier; 2001

[24] Nath RK, Karicherla P, Mahmooduddin F. Shoulder function and anatomy in complete obstetric brachial plexus palsy: long-term improvement after triangle tilt surgery. Child's Nervous System. 2010;26(8):1009-19.

[25] Terzis JK, Papakonstantinou K. Surgical Treatment of Obstetrical Brachial Plexus Paralysis: The Norfolk Experience Seminars in Plastic Surgery. 2004;18(04):359-75.

[26] Abzug JM, Chafetz RS, Gaughan JP, Ashworth S, Kozin SH. Shoulder function after medial approach and derotational humeral osteotomy in patients with brachial plexus birth palsy. Journal of Pediatric Orthopaedics. 2010;30(5):469-74.

[27] Greenhill DA, Trionfo A, Ramsey FV, Kozin SH, Zlotolow DA. Postoperative Loss of Midline Function in Brachial Plexus Birth Palsy. The Journal of Hand Surgery. 2018;43(6).

[28] Clarke HM, Cunis CG. An approach to obstetrical brachial plexus injuries. Hand Clinics. 1995;11(4):563-80.

[29] Bialocerkowski AE, Galea M. Comparison of visual and objective quantification of elbow and shoulder movement in children with obstetric brachial plexus palsy. J Brachial Plex Peripher Nerve Inj. 2006;1(5). DOI: 10.1186/1749-7221-1-5

[30] Bae DS, Waters PM, Zurakowski D: Reliability of three classification systems measuring active motion in brachial plexus birth palsy. J Bone Joint Surg. 2003;85(9):1733-8.

[31] Pondaag W, Malessy MJA. Outcome assessment for Brachial Plexus birth injury. Results from the iPluto world-wide consensus survey. Journal of Orthopaedic Research. 2018;36(9):2533-41.

[32] A Clinicians Guide to the Active Movement Scale (AMS) [Internet]. [cited 2021 May 20]. Available from: https://www.regionvasterbotten.

se/VLL/Filer/AMS%20A%20 Clinicians%20guide%20to%20the%20 Active%20Movement%20Scale.pdf

[33] Michelow BJ, Clarke HM, Curtis CG, et al. The natural history of obstetrical brachial plexus palsy. Plast Reconstr Surg. 1994;93(4):675-680

[34] Greenhill DA, Lukavsky R, Tomlinson-Hansen S, Kozin SH, Zlotolow DA. Relationships Between 3 Classification Systems in Brachial Plexus Birth Palsy. Journal of Pediatric Orthopaedics. 2017;37(6):374-80.

[35] Raimondi P. Evaluation of results in obstetric brachial plexus palsy. The hand. In: International Meeting on Obstetric Brachial Plexus Palsy; 1993; Heerlen, The Netherlands.

[36] Haerle M, Gilbert A. Management of Complete Obstetric Brachial Plexus Lesions. Journal of Pediatric Orthopaedics. 2004;24(2):194-200.

[37] Ruchelsman DE, Pettrone S, Price AE, Grossman JAI. Brachial plexus birth palsy: an overview of early treatment considerations. Bull NYU Hosp Jt Dis. 2009;67(1):83-9.

[38] Sarac C, Duijnisveld BJ, Weide Avan, Schoones JW, Malessy MJA, Nelissen RGHH, et al. Outcome measures used in clinical studies on neonatal brachial plexus palsy: A systematic literature review using the International Classification of Functioning, Disability and Health. Journal of Pediatric Rehabilitation Medicine. 2015;8(3):167-86.

[39] Strömbeck C, Fernell E. Aspects of activities and participation in daily life related to body structure and function in adolescents with obstetrical brachial plexus palsy: a descriptive follow-up study. Acta Paediatrica. 2007;92(6):740-6.

[40] Ho ES, Curtis CG, Clarke HM. The brachial plexus outcome measure: development, internal consistency, and construct validity. Journal of Hand Therapy. 2012;25(4):406-17.

[41] Anguelova GV, Malessy MJA, van Dijk JG. A cross-sectional study of hand sensation in adults with conservatively treated obstetric brachial plexus lesion. Dev Med Child Neurol. 2013;55(3): 257-63.

[42] Johansson GM, Häger CK. A modified standardized nine hole peg test for valid and reliable kinematic assessment of dexterity post-stroke. Journal of NeuroEngineering and Rehabilitation. 2019;16(1).

[43] Immerman I, Alfonso DT, Ramos LE, Grossman LA, Alfornso I, Ditaranto P, Grossman JAI. Hand function in children with an upper brachial plexus birth injury: results of the nine-hole peg test. Developmental Medicine & Child Neurology. 2012; 54(2):166-9.

[44] Chang KW, Justice D, Chung KC, Yang LJ. A systematic review of evaluation methods for neonatal brachial plexus palsy. Journal of Neurosurgery: Pediatrics. 2013;12(4):395-405.

[45] Krumlinde-Sundholm L, Holmefur M, Kottorp A, Eliasson A-C. The Assisting Hand Assessment: current evidence of validity, reliability, and responsiveness to change. Developmental Medicine & Child Neurology. 2007;49(4):259-64.

[46] Hermansson L, Sköld A, Eliasson AC. Bimanual Hand-use in Children with Unilateral Hand Dysfunction– Differences Related to Diagnosis Investigated by the Children's Hand-use Experience Questionnaire. Pediatrics & Therapeutics. 2013;03(04).

[47] Solway S. The DASH outcome measure: user's manual. Toronto: Institute for Work & Health; 2002.

[48] Hudak PL, Amadio PC, Bombardier C, Beaton D, Cole D, Davis A, et al. Development of an upper extremity outcome measure: The DASH (disabilities of the arm, shoulder, and head). American Journal of Industrial Medicine. 1996;29(6):602-8.

[49] Beaton DE, Katz JN, Fossel AH, Wright JG, Tarasuk V, Bombardier C. Measuring the whole or the parts? Validity, reliability, and responsiveness of the Disabilities of the Arm, Shoulder and Hand outcome measure in different regions of the upper extremity. Journal of Hand Therapy. 2001;14(2):128-46.

[50] Quatman-Yates CC, Gupta R, Paterno MV, Schmitt LC, Quatman CE, Ittenbach RF. Internal Consistency and Validity of the QuickDASH Instrument for Upper Extremity Injuries in Older Children. Journal of Pediatric Orthopaedics. 2013;33(8):838-42.

[51] van der Holst M, Geerdink Y, Aarts P, Steenbeek D, Pondaag W, Nelissen RGHH, et al. Hand-Use-at-Home Questionnaire: validity and reliability in children with neonatal brachial plexus palsy or unilateral cerebral palsy. Clinical Rehabilitation. 2018;32(10):1363-73.

[52] Bae DS, Waters PM, Zurakowski D. Correlation of Pediatric Outcomes Data Collection Instrument With Measures of Active Movement in Children With Brachial Plexus Birth Palsy. Journal of Pediatric Orthopaedics. 2008;28(5):584-92.

[53] Daltroy LH, Liang MH, Fossel AH, Goldberg MJ. The POSNA Pediatric Musculoskeletal Functional Health Questionnaire: Report on Reliability, Validity, and Sensitivity to Change. Journal of Pediatric Orthopaedics. 1998;18(5):561-71.

[54] van der Holst M, Steenbeek D, Pondaag W, Nelissen RGHH, Vliet Vlieland TPM. Neonatal Brachial Plexus Palsy in Children Aged 0 to 2.5 Years; Parent-Perceived Family Impact, Quality of Life, and Upper Extremity Functioning. Pediatric Neurology. 2016;62:34-42.

[55] Reinfjell T, Diseth TH, Veenstra M, Vikan A. Measuring health-related quality of life in young adolescents: Reliability and validity in the Norwegian version of the Pediatric Quality of Life Inventory™ 4.0 (PedsQL) generic core scales. Health and Quality of Life Outcomes. 2006;4(1).

[56] Manske MC, Abarca NE, Letzelter JP, James MA. Patient-reported Outcomes Measurement Information System (PROMIS) Scores for Children With Brachial Plexus Birth Injury. Journal of Pediatric Orthopaedics. 2021;41(3):171-6.

[57] Grawburg M, Howe T, Worrall L, Scarinci N. Describing the impact of aphasia on close family members using the ICF framework. Disability and Rehabilitation. 2013;36(14):1184-95.

[58] Basu AP, Pearse J, Kelly S, Wisher V, Kisler J. Early Intervention to Improve Hand Function in Hemiplegic Cerebral Palsy. Frontiers in Neurology. 2015;5.

[59] Steinbok P, Gan PYC, Connolly MB, Carmant L, Barry Sinclair D, Rutka J, et al. Epilepsy surgery in the first 3 years of life: A Canadian survey. Epilepsia. 2009;50(6):1442-9.

[60] Choudhary A, Gulati S, Kabra M, Singh UP, Sankhyan N, Pandey RM, et al. Efficacy of modified constraint induced movement therapy in improving upper limb function in children with hemiplegic cerebral palsy: A randomized controlled trial. Brain and Development. 2013;35(9):870-6.

[61] Keklicek H, Uygur F, Yakut Y. Effects of taping the hand in children with cerebral palsy. Journal of Hand Therapy. 2015;28(1):27-33.

[62] Aroojis A, Sarathy K, Doshi C. Clinical examination of children with cerebral palsy. Indian Journal of Orthopaedics. 2019;53(1):35.

[63] DeMatteo C, Law M, Russell D, Pollock N, Rosenbaum P, Walter S. The Reliability and Validity of the Quality of Upper Extremity Skills Test. Physical & Occupational Therapy In Pediatrics. 1993;13(2):1-18.

[64] Bourke-Taylor H. Melbourne Assessment of Unilateral Upper Limb Function: construct validity and correlation with the Pediatric Evaluation of Disability Inventory. Developmental Medicine & Child Neurology. 2003;45(02).

[65] Mathiowetz V, Federman S, Wiemer D. Box and Block Test of Manual Dexterity: Norms for 6-19 Year Olds. Canadian Journal of Occupational Therapy. 1985;52(5):241-5.

[66] Werning M, Müllner EW, Mlynek G, Dobretzberger V, Djinovic-Carugo K, Baron DM, et al. PKAN neurodegeneration and residual PANK2 activities in patient erythrocytes. Annals of Clinical and Translational Neurology. 2020;7(8):1340-51.

[67] Narayanan UG. Management of Children With Ambulatory Cerebral Palsy. Journal of Pediatric Orthopaedics. 2012;32(Supplement 2).

[68] Debuse D, Brace H. Outcome Measures of Activity for Children With Cerebral Palsy. Pediatric Physical Therapy. 2011;23(3):221-31.

[69] Russo RN, Goodwin EJ, Miller MD, Haan EA, Connell TM, Crotty M. Self-Esteem, Self-Concept, and Quality of Life in Children with Hemiplegic Cerebral Palsy. The Journal of Pediatrics. 2008;153(4).

[70] Christmas PM, Sackley C, Feltham MG, Cummins C. A randomized controlled trial to compare two methods of constraint-induced movement therapy to improve functional ability in the affected upper limb in pre-school children with hemiplegic cerebral palsy: CATCH TRIAL. Clinical Rehabilitation. 2018;32(7):909-18.

[71] Postans N, Wright P, Bromwich W, Wilkinson I, Farmer SE, Swain I. The Combined Effect of Dynamic Splinting and Neuromuscular Electrical Stimulation in Reducing Wrist and Elbow Contractures in Six Children with Cerebral Palsy. Prosthetics & Orthotics International. 2010;34(1):10-9.

[72] James S, Ziviani J, Boyd R. A systematic review of activities of daily living measures for children and adolescents with cerebral palsy. Developmental Medicine & Child Neurology. 2013;56(3):233-44.

[73] Law M, Baptiste S, McColl MA, Opzoomer A, Polatajko H, Pollock N. The Canadian Occupational Performance Measure: An Outcome Measure for Occupational Therapy. Canadian Journal of Occupational Therapy. 1990;57(2):82-7.

[74] Tofani M, Castelli E, Sabbadini M, Berardi A, Murgia M, Servadio A, et al. Examining Reliability and Validity of the Jebsen-Taylor Hand Function Test Among Children With Cerebral Palsy. Perceptual and Motor Skills. 2020;127(4):684-97.

[75] Law M, Baptiste S, McColl MA, Opzoomer A, Polatajko H, Pollock N. The Canadian Occupational Performance Measure: An Outcome Measure for Occupational Therapy. Canadian Journal of Occupational Therapy. 1990;57(2):82-7.

[76] Cardenas A, Warner D, Switzer L, Graham TCN, Cimolino G, Fehlings D. Inpatient Exergames for Children with Cerebral Palsy following Lower

Extremity Orthopedic Surgery: A Feasibility Study. Developmental Neurorehabilitation. 2021;24(4):230-6.

[77] Ryll UC, Krumlinde-Sundholm L, Verhage CH, Sicola E, Sgandurra G, Bastiaenen CHG, et al. Predictive validity of the Hand Assessment for Infants in infants at risk of unilateral cerebral palsy. Developmental Medicine & Child Neurology. 2020;63(4):436-43.

[78] Arnould C. Practical Considerations of the Both Hands Assessment (BoHA): A commentary on "Development and Validation of the Both Hands Assessment for Children with Bilateral Cerebral Palsy." Physical & Occupational Therapy In Pediatrics. 2018;38(2):127-9.

[79] Romeo DM, Brogna C, Quintiliani M, Baranello G, Pagliano E, Casalino T, et al. Sleep disorders in children with cerebral palsy: neurodevelopmental and behavioral correlates. Sleep Medicine. 2014;15(2):213-8.

[80] Morgan C, Novak I, Dale RC, Guzzetta A, Badawi N. Single blind randomised controlled trial of GAME (Goals - Activity - Motor Enrichment) in infants at high risk of cerebral palsy. Research in Developmental Disabilities. 2016;55:256-67.

[81] Bjornson KF, Zhou C, Stevenson R, Christakis DA. Capacity to Participation in Cerebral Palsy: Evidence of an Indirect Path Via Performance. Archives of Physical Medicine and Rehabilitation. 2013;94(12):2365-72.

Chapter 7

# Factors of Cortical Plasticity in Brachial Plexus Injury

*Jennifer Reinsch, Anna Zdunczyk, Tarik Alp Sargut, Maren Denker, Melina Engelhardt, Peter Vajkoczy, Thomas Picht and Nora Dengler*

## Abstract

Cortical plasticity is the brain's capability of decoding new information through growth and reorganization over our whole life spam. It is the basis for good outcomes after reinnervation and for rehabilitation of adult and obstetric brachial plexus injury. Knowledge about cortical reorganization is crucial to reconstructive surgeons and physiotherapists that aim to give their patients a reasonable prognosis. This chapter intends to present and summarize the current literature on how to detect and quantify cortical plasticity and how research on factors that influence cortical plasticity, mainly in relation to peripheral nerve and more precise brachial plexus injury progresses. Peculiarities of adult and obstetric brachial plexus injuries and their treatment are given. We present techniques that visualize and quantify cortical plasticity with focus on functional imaging like fMRI and nTMS as well as molecular aspects. Future research is needed to understand mechanisms of how molecular changes on a synaptic level of a neuron influence the macroscopic plasticity, to improve rehabilitative resources, to understand the exact prognostic value of nTMS in brachial plexus injury and to investigate the therapeutic capability of rTMS.

**Keywords:** cortical plasticity, cortical reorganization, adult brachial plexus injury, obstetric brachial plexus injuries, nTMS, motor cortex, peripheral nerve lesion

## 1. Introduction

Cortical plasticity in general is the ability of neuronal tissue to adapt to changing requirements. It may either be a regular mechanism in physiological tissue, or it appears after a central or peripheral injury. After brachial plexus injury, for instance, the respective cortical area of the denervated peripheral nerves gets reorganized after a certain time. Neighboring cortical areas migrate in the direction of the newly formed "black whole", until they occupy the area.

This chapter aims to give insights on how cortical plasticity may be detected and quantified, why it is important for the outcome of patients with peripheral nerve injury and how this may impact outcome prediction and outcome modification in our patients.

Treatment of peripheral nerve injury and more precise brachial plexus injury includes rehabilitation as well as reconstructive surgery. Reconstructive surgery is



IntechOpen

composed of the restoration of nerve function by nerve graft or nerve transfer or secondary reconstructive techniques that may include tendon or muscle transfers.

Nerve graft means to bridge the proximal and distal end of the affected peripheral nerve with a donor nerve.

Nerve transfer is a technique where a functional donor nerve keeps its proximal connection to the CNS and gets transferred on the affected nerve with its distal end.

Tendon transfer means the transfer of one functional tendon on a second tendon whose muscle is paralytic due to a spinal or peripheral nerve injury.

Muscle transfer is the removal of an autologous muscle and the subsequent implantation on another part of the body to improve functions after nerve injury, for example.

Static techniques offer some benefit, when dynamic procedures cannot be performed. An example would be the glenohumeral fusion after axillary nerve injury.

A major question in past and future research is: what happens with the cortical representation of muscle and nerve function after reconstructive surgery and which associated factors may impact patient's outcome?

It is of high importance to the surgeon to be able to give his or her patient a realistic prognosis of the degree of recovery after surgery. For this purpose, a certain knowledge of how cortical reorganization influences the prognosis of the surgical treatment is essential. Because of that, this chapter dives deeper into some surgical techniques to help answering questions like why, for instance, an intercostal nerve as donor leads to a better outcome in the biceps muscle concerning levels of strength, compared to the hypoglossal nerve.

The passage which follows gives an overview of the most important imaging techniques, which are essential to measure cortical plasticity in humans.

The main body of our chapter thereafter summarizes promising scientific work on cortical plasticity in peripheral nerve injury in animals and humans and tries to answer the main questions of this chapter mentioned above. Naturally, relatively macroscopic changes in motor cortex underlie changes on a molecular basis. The following passage will provide the basic approaches, as well as recent developments in the field of synaptic plasticity, as they are a prerequisite for the understanding of cortical plasticity in the future.

In summary, this chapter gives an introduction in adult and obstetric brachial plexus injury. It gives definitions, and traces different types, surgical treatments, and outcome. Next, two excellent imaging methods, fMRI and nTMS will be introduced.

In the main part, cortical plasticity will be disentangled, progress in research in animals and humans concerning cortical plasticity in peripheral neve injuries, different types of CNS pathways involved in that, and a short introduction to the molecular background, as mentioned above, are given.

To conclude this, future prospects and suggestions for further research are shown, a conclusion will finally sum it up.

## 2. Adult brachial plexus injury

### 2.1 Definitions and types

Although adult brachial plexus injuries are relatively rare, they are nonetheless a highly traumatic injury to a patient and can cause severe disability and pain. A common cause is, above all, high-velocity trauma caused by car or motorcycle accident, which are sudden events leading to lasting physical and psychological handicaps.

Anatomically and clinically, we can subclassify brachial plexus injuries in upper and lower trunk lesions, resulting in different deficiencies. Upper trunk brachial plexus injuries (C5-C6 roots) appear as a loss of shoulder abduction, external rotation, elbow flexion, and forearm supination [1]. In comparison to this, lower trunk brachial plexus injuries (C7, C8, Th1) typically lead to a loss of elbow extension and deficits in finger and wrist movement. The extent or degree of nerve injury may be classified according to Sunderland. The classification specifies five degrees of nerve damage. The first one is neurapraxia, which is an impermanent loss of motor and sensory function due to persistent pressure or overstretching. Degree two to four describe different stages of axonotmesis, grade five stands for neurotmesis (see 2.2) [2].

### 2.2 Surgical treatment and outcome

For the treatment of brachial plexus injuries, in general, a balanced estimation has to be made in terms of time to wait for spontaneous recovery, which can occur in mild lesions with axonotmesis [3]. Axonotmesis describes the transection of an axon with preserved nerve sheath.

On the other hand, neurotmesis, which describes the rupture of the axon and up to all surrounding structures, or avulsion of the nerve root from the spinal cord will most likely not lead to spontaneous recovery [3]. In this case, a variety of surgical repairing techniques has been developed to reconstruct nerve function.

Basically, there are multiple ways of reconnecting muscle tissue to the central nervous system.

A nerve graft or nerve transplantation is an established way to bridge proximal and distal ends of an injured nerve. An example for a nerve graft would be to bypass an injured accessory nerve by use of smaller donors like the sural or auricularis magnus nerve.

Then there is nerve transfer. In this procedure, a functional donor nerve is sacrificed and gets connected to the affected muscle or the transected distal part of the injured nerve. In terms of upper brachial plexus injuries, Leechavengvuongs and Oberlin transfers are common and successful procedures, which are going to be explained in detail in the next passage.

There are further techniques, like tendon transfer, which is the transfer of one functional tendon on a second tendon whose muscle is paralytic due to a peripheral nerve injury. An example would be a tendon transfer for drop foot correction.

Muscle transfer is the removal of an autologous muscle and the subsequent implantation on another part of the body to improve functions after nerve injury, for example.

For the upper brachial plexus injury, the restoration of elbow flexion should be given the highest priority. Secondly, shoulder abduction, followed by external rotation are important functions.

Concerning elbow flexion, in general, nerve grafting led to better outcomes compared to nerve transfers. But taken alone the Oberlin transfer as an independent procedure, its outcomes are better than nerve grafting, nerve transfers or combined techniques [1].

In upper brachial plexus injury, the failure of the musculocutaneous nerve leads to a deficiency in elbow flexion due to a disconnection to the biceps muscle. In the Oberlin procedure, one fascicle of the ulnar nerve is being sacrificed as a donor nerve for a nerve graft to the musculocutaneous nerve close to the access to the biceps muscle. A fast motor recovery is being observed due to the close transfer to the muscle [4].

Another option is the phrenic or intercostal nerve transfer to the musculocutaneous nerve, which will be discussed as a well-researched example further below.

Regarding shoulder abduction, nerve transfer was significantly more successful than nerve grafting or combined techniques [1]. A disruption of the axillary nerve leads to abductor weakness in the deltoid muscle. The Leechavengvuongs transfer uses one radial nerve branch to be transferred onto the axillary nerve to restore abductor function [5, 6].

For the lower brachial plexus injury, the reinnervation of the median nerve for digital sensibility and forearm flexor function, and the radial nerve for the extension of the elbow, wrist and fingers are higher priorities, compared to the ulnar nerve, because the chance of recovery is lowest here. This is also the reason for usually taking the ulnar nerve as a nerve graft, besides the more commonly used sural nerve, to restore more important functions.

All in all, it is still not clarified why one repairing technique is better than the other in different settings. Presumably, the superiority of nerve transfers in some occasions is based on a combination of different influential factors. A shorter distance for nerve regeneration, only one suture junction and a vascularized donor nerve can be some reasons [1].

A deeper knowledge of how cortical plasticity influences the progress of reorganization of the affected motor areas is therefore an essential prerequisite for a satisfying outcome. What are requirements for a successful reinnervation, concerning the right choice of donor nerve, surgical treatment and rehabilitation procedure on the cortical level? How do other factors, like the age, influence plasticity?

To clarify this later, an overview on obstetric brachial plexus injury follows.

## 3. Obstetric brachial plexus injury

### 3.1 Definitions, incidence and types

The obstetric brachial plexus injury (OBPI) is a birth trauma, which may be associated with complicated childbirth. Injuries are more common in the upper brachial plexus (50% C5 and C6, 25% C5 to C7) or the panplexus (20%), rarely in the lower brachial plexus (2%) alone.

With one shoulder blocked by the mother's symphysis and the head already born, the injury is usually caused by tension on the neck and shoulder region, which can lead to a rupture of the neural structures mentioned above. This can occur during natural and vacuum deliveries.

With an incidence of about 0.1 to 3 per 1000 live births, it is a relatively rare injury, which nonetheless influences the child's life and can causes severe disability and pain.

In [7], shoulder dystocia has been identified as the main risk factor for obstetric brachial plexus injury. Others are an exceptionally high birth weight > 4.5 kilograms, breech delivery, instrumented delivery, maternal diabetes and other minor factors. In contrast to that, delivery by cesarean section and twin birth count as protective factors. In addition, there are also references mentioning an intrauterine genesis of obstetric brachial plexus injury [8]. It is important to mention that the majority of cases did not have any risk factors.

The severity of the injury is based on the degree of damage caused to the neurons. Like in adult brachial plexus injury, neurapraxia (reversible stretching) and axonotmesis have a higher chance of recovery, compared to neurotmesis, which is the rupture of the whole axon and up to all its surrounding structures. Avulsion from the spinal cord does not really have a chance for spontaneous improvement.

### 3.2 Surgical treatment and outcome

Spontaneous recovery occurred in 70 to 80% of all obstetric brachial plexus injuries, the other cases needed treatment due to incomplete motor recovery or an otherwise unsatisfying outcome.

On conservative treatment, no randomized controlled studies could be found. An improved outcome could not be found for primary surgical treatment in comparison to non-operative management. Nonetheless, surgical management was superior to conservative management in severe cases. In those children, primary surgical management led to a better outcome compared to secondary surgical repair, but still improved motor recovery. Overall, treatment of these children required a multidisciplinary team, as still 25% of the patients are affected by permanent disability [8].

Surgical treatment consists of direct suturing or the surgical techniques mentioned above. For minor injuries, exploration of the affected plexus parts and resection of neuroma are treatment options. Primary reconstruction of the obstetric brachia plexus injury leads to a satisfying outcome in terms of motor and sensitivity of hand and elbow for most patients. A second surgical intervention is sometimes needed to improve motor functions in wrist and shoulder [9, 10].

When we compare the outcome of surgical treatments of brachial plexus injury in adults and infants, the second group gains a much better hand function in the long term. This could be justified by the cause of the injury: In adults, this is usually a high-velocity trauma, like a car or motorcycle accident, compared to the forcefully overstretch of the head-shoulder region during birth in infants. On one hand, a worse outcome for hand function could be influenced by other severe injuries in the musculotosceletal area in adults [11]. On the other hand, the major factor influencing cortical plasticity, and therefore the motor outcome, is age, which will be discussed below (5.4).

## 4. Functional imaging methods

### 4.1 fMRI

fMRI (functional magnetic resonance imaging) is a variation of MRI (magnetic resonance imaging). It detects changes in tissue perfusion in different brain regions, generated by a changing energy consumption of active nerve cells.

The BOLD (Blood-Oxygenation-Level Dependent)-Effect is a basic principle, which the fMRI is based on. It depends on the presence of oxygenated hemoglobin, which has no magnetic characteristics, compared to deoxygenated blood, which is paramagnetic. This leads to the appearance of a magnetic field, which results in a changing of rotation properties in hydrogen protons.

Briefly, neuronal activation leads to a hemodynamic response in the respective area, which results in a different spinning behavior of protons and therefore to the identification of active areas on the resulting image. It is important to note that this reaction is an indirect measure of neural activity and underlies a delay of about five seconds, which lowers the temporal resolution of this imaging method. In terms of spatial resolution, compared to other imaging techniques, fMRI provides comparatively good outcomes.

Neuronal activity can either be evocated deliberately through tasks carried out by the patient during the measurement, or passively as a resting state fMRI, which shows the patient's baseline bold variance.

Apart from the good spatial resolution, fMRI has the advantages of not using ionizing radiation and being painless for the patient. Also, it covers the whole brain, including deeply localized brain structures.

fMRI can be used to detect sensorimotor, as well as language and visual cortices, but its lack of specificity and sensitivity prevents it from becoming a gold standard for the identification of such cortical regions. Apart from that, it might not always represent real neural activity, as the signal changes with modified vascularization. Finally, the MRI being a relatively loud imaging technique, makes it not the ideal method for examining speech and language functions as it influences its own results [12].

### 4.2 nTMS

Transcranial magnetic stimulation (TMS) is a non-invasive diagnostic tool to map eloquent areas for motor and speech function on the cortical surface . A figure of eight shaped magnetic coil elicits an electric impulse on the patient's head surface hereby leading to a depolarization of cortical neurons. Navigated TMS (nTMS) uses a high resolution T1 navigation sequence to generate an anatomical model of the patient's head. By navigating the stimulation coil and a head tracker positioned on the subject's forehead a high anatomical precision in cortical mapping can be achieved. Motor responses are recorded by a free running EMG recorded surface electrodes on the corresponding muscles.

A big advantage of the nTMS technique is the possibility to navigate accurately and individualized, but non-invasive.

During the measurement two objects are being located constantly in a 3D space: First, information about the position of the patient's head, in case of movement, has to be transmitted to the system. For this case, a so called "head tracker" is fixed on the forehead, which is in constant connection to an optical positioning sensor. Secondly, the 3D position of the coil and intensity of the resulting magnetic field has to be tracked simultaneously to allow optical orientation and therefore precise stimulation. Here, a coil tracker transmits information about orientation, location and tilting as relative coordinates to the positioning sensor.

The examiner connects the MRI scan and the real head through the use of a digitizer pen at the beginning of a session by pointing given anatomical landmarks on both the MRI scan and the head. Algorithms then link the scan to the patient's head coordinates and enable the examiner to see a real time e-field, which is dependent on the position of the coil on an MRI 3D-model, on the nTMS system display. Apart from those devices, nTMS hardware also includes a stimulator. It produces the output pulse given by the nTMS software.

Furthermore, an EMG is attached on the side of the examination chair to record motor evoked potentials (MEPs). MEPs are displayed on a free running EMG on the display next to the 3D MRI model of the subject's head. They are synchronous to each stimulation and determine the color of the stimulation spot on the MRI, which depends on the amplitude of the MEP. Lastly, a foot pedal is there to apply stimuli and adjust intensity easily without having to move one hand from the coil (**Figure 1**).

For motor mappings, a stimulation along the central sulcus according to the localization of the homunculus is performed. A few of the important parameters of TMS are the Center of Gravity, which resembles the amplitude-weighted position of the determined muscle on the motor map. The Motor threshold is the minimum TMS intensity necessary to induce a motor-evoked potential from a specific muscle. It refers to the inherent excitability [13]. Especially for the hand and arm motor area, stimulation of the central sulcus, precentral gyrus and sulcus and postcentral

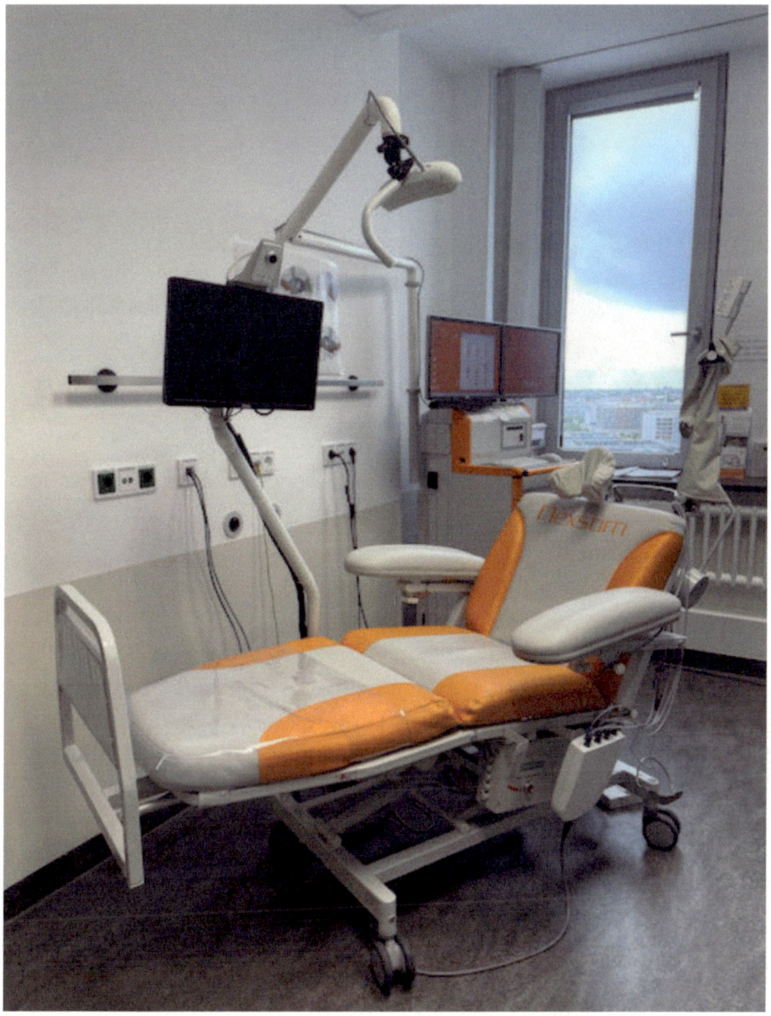

**Figure 1.**
*TMS hardware.*

sulcus is recommended (please see [12] for more information on how to perform an nTMS session) (**Figure 2**).

In summary, nTMS is a noninvasive motor mapping technique that allows us to find the precise cortical location of motor or language functions in real time. Clinical applications include in particular the preoperative mapping of language regions and motor mapping in the management of peri-Rolandic tumors to locate the pyramidal tract [12].

As for the limitations of this technique, the first point to mention is precision. A study [14] estimates the spatial accuracy being better than 5 mm. As the tolerance for registration is limited to 2-3 mm, one has to keep in mind that brain and surrounding tissue can undergo changes due to neoplastic activities or intraoperative movement.

Secondly, the magnetic field itself can be a limitation, as magnetic pulses sometimes spread into subcortical white matter tracts. The activation of neurons situated there can be misinterpreted as motor function.

Thirdly, some basic parameters in both motor and language mapping are not yet investigated sufficiently enough, so that small adjustments in intensity and timing can have a bigger impact on the measurement than it is known yet.

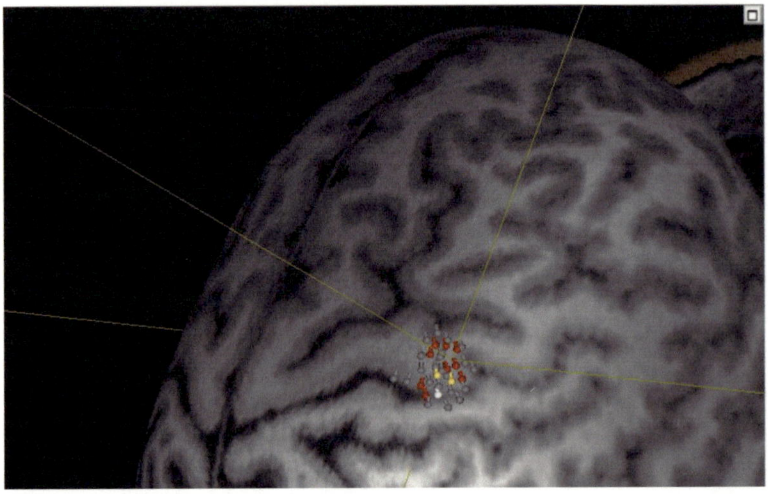

**Figure 2.**
*Example of stimulation results around hand area.*

A comparison of the two functional imaging techniques described above includes advantages and disadvantages in terms of temporal and spatial resolution, accurateness and feasibility. fMRI has the disadvantage of measuring neural activity indirectly through the product of three consecutive metabolic reactions, which delays the output by several seconds. In temporal considerations, nTMS is more accurate, as it more or less only takes the conduction velocity of the respective nerve between in- and output. For spatial resolution, fMRI has the advantage of reaching deeper brain regions on the one hand, but is not able to detect white matter connections, on the other hand. Compared to that, nTMS only has a magnetic field strong enough to reach a depth of two to three centimeters. Regarding certain artifacts, nTMS is resistant to abnormal vasculature, whereas fMRI gets affected by that. Although there are some contraindications for nTMS, such as aneurysm clips and deep brain stimulators, they do not pose a risk for the patient, as they would do in an MRI. Also not unimportant is the factor of patient participation. As for motor mappings, no patient participation is required, although sessions can get really long for patients, as well as quite painful during some measurements due to high stimulation intensities. fMRI on the other side can cause claustrophobia, but is usually not painful. In terms of accuracy, nTMS produces motor maps with the highest concordance rates with intraoperative DES motor maps [15].

As both of these techniques have their strengths, it is important to know the indications and to pick the most suitable functional imaging method individually.

### 4.3 Other measuring techniques

Further measuring techniques, apart from fMRI and nTMS, are summarized in **Table 1**. A short description, strengths and weaknesses are displayed to gain a quick overview. For the sake of completeness and comparability, fMRI and nTMS are again included.

It can be suggested that a multi-modal approach as a combination of some of these techniques could be most effective to gain an integrated picture of cortical plasticity [17]. For instance, it would make sense to combine techniques with the advantage of being able to measure with both a high temporal and spatial resolution.

| Measuring technique | How it works | What is measured | Strengths | Weaknesses |
|---|---|---|---|---|
| **fMRI** | MRI + BOLD effect (see above) | Sctive areas through changes in tissue perfusion | Reaches deeply located brain regions; non-invasive | Temporal resolution; indirect measurement; contraindications |
| **nTMS** | Magnetic coil induces electric field on cortex (see above) | In general: representation of a muscle on motor cortex (for motor mappings) | Temporal resolution; no patient participation required | Spatial resolution: only cortex (+ close underlying structures) → bidimensional |
| **Cortical stimulation mapping (DES)** | Current causes reversible lesion in small area | In general: representation of one or more muscles on motor cortex | Gold standard: temporal and spatial resolution | Craniotomy required |
| **Magneto-encephalography (MEG)** [16] | Estimation of magnetic field generated by electric currents in brain | Direct measurement of sensimotor areas | Temporal resolution | MEG device expensive → not as common |
| **Positron emission tomography (PET)** | Radioactive tracer accumulates in metabolically active regions | Active areas due to a high metabolism | Spatial resolution | Temporal resolution, radiopharmaceutical injection |
| **Electro-encephalography (EEG)** | Electrical potential changes of pyramidal cells displayed as curves | Electrical potential changes over area of a few centimeters | Temporal resolution | Spatial resolution (centimeters) |

**Table 1.**
*Overview of cortical plasticity measuring techniques.*

For rehabilitation, [18] combined EEG and rTMS to gain a real time picture of the excitability brain state to control the efficiency of cortical plasticity induced by rTMS, to name only one example.

## 5. Cortical plasticity after peripheral nerve injuries

### 5.1 Introduction and definition

It is an established opinion in neuroscience for several decades now that the brain is not a rigid and inflexible organ, but highly capable of decoding new information through growth and reorganization over our whole life spam. All cortical areas are able to process practiced movement or sensory experience, which called Cortical Plasticity. It is the ability to increase cortex area that represents a certain peripheral input which is proportionally most used.

To understand the background of cortical plasticity, a closer look has to be taken on molecular mechanisms underlying this phenomenon. Already in 1949, Donald Hebb postulated that "When an axon of cell A is near enough to excite B and repeatedly or persistently takes part in firing it, some growth process or metabolic change takes place in one or both cells such that A's efficiency, as one of the cells firing B, is increased" [19]. Several molecular mechanisms, including long-term potentiation and long-term depression, underlie this feedback loop, which will be presented below (5.5).

The same basic principles that underlie encoding of practice or experience can be detected in cortical reorganization following lesions of the central nervous system. Although a lot of literature can be found on that, the consequences of cortical reorganization after peripheral denervation and, subsequently, after surgical reinnervation, are still not well investigated and understood, especially humans. Some findings in the field of motor cortex reorganization come from fMRI and TMS studies that were made after peripheral nerve injury or amputation. In contrast to that, there are already interesting findings in animal research.

### 5.2 Cortical plasticity in animals

Cortical plasticity following peripheral nerve injuries has been investigated in animals, especially in mice, rats and primates.

Merzenich et al. [20] and Jenkins et al. [21] are often-quoted articles from the 1980's. In [20], the median nerve was transected and ligated in adult monkeys, which lead to the inability of flexing the affected hand's first three fingers. Through microelectrode mapping several months after the transection of the nerve, one found the former representative areas of the affected fingers occupied by expanded representations of surrounding skin fields. Large new representative fields of finger four and five, as well as of the dorsal parts of fingers one, two, and three were found. Some fields only expanded, some other moved completely into the former areas of the denervated fingers. The topographic order of the remaining fingers was reported to be regular, the size of the expanded or "new" areas approximately correlated with the size of the original ones.

It could be observed that synaptic connections between motor cortex and somatic musculature are continually reshaped in young and adult animals. In terms of timing, it has been found that synaptic changes in motor cortex start developing at most hours after the peripheral nerve transection, and continue their formation at least for months.

Donoghue et al. [22] unmasked latent intracortical connections by pharmacologically blocking intracortical inhibition via GABA antagonists. Thereby, preexisting excitatory connections inside the motor cortex were revealed. In this experiment, a peripheral nerve of adult rats got transected and simultaneously blocked by GABA on the cortex level, and within a few hours, in the cortical territory of the affected body part, movements represented in adjacent primary motor cortex areas were evoked. Due to this study, one can assume the existence of fibers in healthy subjects which can form a possible basic structure of plasticity after peripheral nerve injury.

The same group gave another example [23] of rapid motor cortex reorganization after motor nerve transection in rats. With the help of maps made by intracortical electrical stimulation, comparisons between healthy rats and animals with a facial nerve lesion showed a shift from vibrissae to forelimb representational areas within hours after facial nerve transection. This again shows a continuous reshaping of synaptic relations between motor cortex and somatic musculature in adult mammals.

Apart from changes in the motor cortex representation within hours after a lesion, [24] found long-term patterns of reorganization after lesions set between one week and four months before. Again, with the help of maps made by intracortical electrical stimulation, comparisons between healthy rats and rats with a facial nerve lesion and, this time, rats with a forelimb amputation, showed an enlarged area representing the forelimb and eye/eyelid output for facial nerve transected animals and an increase of the area for shoulder movements for the limb amputated animals. As the extent of some representations of healthy musculature in both experimental conditions increased, it can be concluded that M1 output relationships with target muscles reorganize in response to nerve injury in adult animals with a long-lasting effect, considering the rat's life span of about two years.

### 5.3 Cortical plasticity in humans

Cortical plasticity following nerve transection has been investigated in humans, too, whereas literature lacks in studies about cortical reorganization after nerve transfer or nerve graft. In contrast to animal studies, imaging methods like direct cortical stimulation can hardly be used in human subjects concerning the observation of cortical reorganization after peripheral nerve injuries. Therefore, the above-mentioned methods of fMRI, nTMS, as well as magnetoencephalography (MEG), and positron emission tomography (PET) can be used with all their advantages and disadvantages. As mentioned above, TMS provides detailed motor maps, fMRI provides good spatial resolution, MEG provides almost real-time temporal resolution, in return. A well-chosen combination of those techniques and derivates, like fiber tracking, is essential to study cortical reorganization.

A look on different factors that determine outcome after surgical reinnervation shows that there are multiple criterions on which a successful intervention depends:

In the first place, there is the distance between the cortical areas of donor and receptor neuron. A mentioned previously, latent intracortical connections could possibly be more distinct between areas that are located closer to each other on the motor cortex. For example, in some cases, the hypoglossal nerve has been used for a musculocutaneous transfer. Outcomes had been poor, because cortical motor areas of both nerves are distantly located. In contrast to that, a hypoglossal-facial nerve transfer shows better results, probably due to a closer location. Another good example would be the success rate of the transfer of an intercostal to the musculocutaneous nerve: The two nerves, though not being connected to the same body part, probably share preexisting connections, because of body posture control being an essential requirement for elbow flexion.

Secondly, a presence or absence of lowly active interneural connections are also likely to determine the outcome, which resembles the first point. Immediately after deafferentation, unmasking of those fibers is probably based on the reduction of GABAergic inhibition of neighboring neurons. This theory could be supported by the detection of reduced GABA-staining at least in somatosensory cortex [25]. Also, the unmasking of previously "silent" thalamocortical projections could play a role in the immediate events taking place after a nerve transection.

Thirdly, as a main principle, the recovery of gross movements, like elbow flexion, succeeds more often than that of finer movements, like finger or hand movements. This fact could be based on the large area the hand occupies on motor cortex, which is not so easy to be supported by enough axon donors surgically.

Fourthly, the long-term outcome depends on rehabilitation, which should start early after intervention, include many repetitions and last two years minimum. Additionally, sensory input is important for a motoric rehabilitation, so ideally, sufficient sensory function should be ensured previously.

Finally, outcome clearly depends on the age at transection and on the degree of injury, naturally. As above-mentioned, the treatment of neonatal brachial plexus injuries has excellent results, which can be reasoned by a better axonal regenerative capacity, but also by the shorter distances from the muscle to the brachial plexus. In summary, two basic rules for successful reinnervation could be determined: A close cortical location of the donor and acceptor nerve region and similar motor control pathways, as well as the existence of (latent) connections between them [13, 26].

For studying effects of peripheral reinnervation on the cortex, fMRI might not be the ideal tool, because it shows neural activity related to input and intracortical processing, rather than output signals. In patients with reinnervated biceps muscle, the M1 area representing the biceps of both affected and contralateral side showed no difference between them neither in the number of active pixels, nor in the mean value of their activations. So, although both areas seemed to activate the biceps muscle of the respective side, the affected muscle could not have been reached by it [27, 28].

In contrast to that, TMS studies showed that a lateral shift of the intercostal nerve area takes place shortly after the intercostal-musculocutaneous nerve transfer. Little by little, this area conquers the former musculocutaneous area on motor cortex. At the end of the process, it occupies the physiologic biceps area [27]. In another TMS study, after the above-mentioned intervention, the cortical area of the biceps of the affected arm was smaller and less excitable than the contralateral one. But also, the newly-shifted former intercostal nerve area of the affected side has been found occupying the former biceps side, which is a similar finding to the experiment above [29].

Apart from diagnostics, repetitive transcranial magnetic stimulation (rTMS) is used as a therapeutic tool. Recently, level A evidence was reached in the treatment of neuropathic pain, depression, and for hand motor recovery in the post-acute stage of stroke.

On healthy subjects, TMS was applied with the help of closed-loop stimulation. Passively moving their hand via brain-machine-interface, subjects activated TMS stimulation of their motor cortex. This synchronized coupled stimulation led to the recruitment of additional corticospinal pathways [30].

Additionally, also in a healthy subject, TMS in combination with a brain-machine interface increased the mean motor evoked potential (MEP). Compared to that, the mean MEP could not be increased in a patient with ischemic hemiplegia for five years with this experimental treatment [31].

All in all, experience should be gained on if and how (reinnervated) peripheral nerve injuries could possibly be treated with TMS.

### 5.4 Different types of CNS pathways involved

As mentioned above, denervation of the musculocutaneous nerve can be reinnervated by a nerve transfer of an intercostal nerve. As intercostal nerves were previously connected to muscles in charge of respiration and posture control, patients are postoperatively able to move their biceps muscle through inhaling. It can be observed that, after months, patients are able to flex their elbow directly, which means without the "trick" of breathing. A TMS-study examined this condition. Patients were stimulated during breathing, rest and voluntary contraction of the biceps. In contrast to shortly after the reinnervation, MEPs were highest for the voluntary contraction, compared to the muscle activity during respiration and rest. That implies that a shift must have been taken place, where the cortical area once responsible for breathing and posture control now enables a muscle of the arm to volitionally contract. Still, typical respiratory EMG activity could be observed in subjects [32]. This is only one example of many, but the question is: Why and how does this change of cortical connectivity happen?

First, the above-mentioned study named the formation of new direct connections between the cortical intercostal nerve and musculocutaneous nerve area. Through TMS, a lateral shift of the intercostal nerve area in the direction of the biceps area could be observed. In the end, it occupied the original biceps area.

Secondly, axonal sprouting could be one of many, probably colluding, factors contributing to cortical plasticity.

Thirdly, as already mentioned above, the cortex most likely contains a large network of partly inactive, inhibited fibers, which gets stronger once another inhibiting structure fails due to denervation and serves as a matrix or skeletal structure for new connections to build on. These preexisting latent networks are probably stronger between areas with a similar function or movements often done simultaneously, for example stretching of the elbow and stretching of the wrist. Latent connections between the biceps and intercostal muscles could preexist due to the need of posture control during (powerful) biceps contraction.

Below, a table summarizes the above-mentioned factors influencing cortical plasticity after peripheral nerve lesion. These factors should always be kept in mind when planning a reconstructive surgery (**Table 2**).

### 5.5 Molecular background

Changes in synaptic plasticity seem to be the basic principle underlying cortical plasticity. To study motor cortex reorganization, e.g., after brachial plexus injury, it is crucial to understand how a change in peripheral input modifies patterns of neuronal firing.

The above-mentioned rule of Donald Hebb or, in short, "Neurons that fire together, wire together", serves as a basic principle underlying synaptic plasticity. Although not much was known then about the molecular background of synaptic firing, Hebb's rule was experimentally confirmed over the years. In general, high-frequency stimulation induces synaptic potentiation, whereas long lasting, low-frequency stimulation induces synaptic depression. These changes in synaptic strength can last for a short or longer (several minutes) period of time. In this case, the change in firing frequency is called long-term potentiation (LTP) or long-term depression (LTD). Very long-lasting firing patterns depend on a change in protein synthesis. These changes in synaptic activity can be illustrated with the help of differential equations, which shall not be discussed here [41].

| Factor | Short explanation | References |
|---|---|---|
| Time between injury and repair | Balance between waiting for spontaneous recovery and worsening requirements for surgical repair | [33] |
| Distance between cortical areas of donor and receptor nerve | The smaller the distance, the higher the chance of an increase in connectivity between areas | [26] |
| Rough vs. fine movement reconstruction | Rough movement seems to be easier to reconstruct | [34] |
| | | [35] |
| Lowly active interneural connections | Lowly active interneural connections are masked and detectable whilst increasing their activity after failure of overlying fibers | [22] |
| | | [32] |
| Trauma | In general, "black holes", as results from brain trauma, seem to be occupied by neighboring areas | [20, 21] |
| | | [23, 24] |
| Age | The younger the brain, the more potential for cortical plasticity | [36] |
| | | [37] |
| | | [38] |
| | | [39] |
| Rehabilitation | Starting early preoperatively and lasting at least two years | [40] |

**Table 2.**
*Summary of factors influencing cortical plasticity after peripheral nerve lesion, modified according to Socolovsky et al. [26].*

In the rodent barrel cortex, where sensory input of whisker movement gets processed, information of each single whisker is transmitted to a specific neuronal cell cluster. It has been found out that cutting every but a single one whisker induces the building of further connections between these cell clusters in the form of LTP. Shortly after cutting the whiskers, a few sensorial inputs lead to an increased number of N-methyl-D-aspartate (NMDA) receptors in the postsynaptic membrane, which lead to an increase in glutamate transmission and thus to a higher information transmission. Interestingly, after further usage of the single whisker, further synaptic plasticity gets induced by an increased number of metabotropic glutamate (mGlu) receptors in the postsynaptic membrane, which probably leads to a long-lasting increase of AMPA receptor. This enables the cell of a higher calcium influx, which forms the basic molecular background of LTPs [42, 43]. After all, LTP is now believed to be a more complex, multicomponent process, that is not yet fully understood.

Recent models however have revealed a variety of other forms of plasticity in neocortex. Plasticity of intrinsic excitability, plasticity of GABAergic circuits, homeostatic synaptic scaling and metaplasticity are the most important. As all of these models are based on physiological neuronal tissue, lesion-induced plasticity can possibly depend on partly different mechanisms.

Plasticity of intrinsic excitability is a neuron's electrical excitability, which is influenced by the number of receptors and distribution and number of ion channels that determine the electrical potential of the neuron. A little neglected earlier in synaptic plasticity research, it nowadays seems to play an important role on the microscopic level of cortical plasticity [44].

Plasticity of GABAergic circuits, as mentioned above, is believed to also play an important role in synaptic plasticity in controlling a balance of excitation and inhibition. Inhibitor cells, too, have the ability of the production of LTP and LTD. GABAergic neurons are associated of being one of the regulatory elements in maintaining homeostatic plasticity. For instance, a twenty-four-hour continuous whisker stimulation decreases cortical activity due to overstimulation, which is a homeostatic mechanism based on the inhibitory activity of GABAergic cells [45].

Homeostatic synaptic scaling is caused by decreased neuronal firing activity, which leads to a decreased somatic calcium concentration. This lowers the amount of activated Calcium/calmodulin-dependent protein kinase type IV (CaMKIV), which then activates the transcription of a "scaling factor". After this, alpha-amino-3-hydroxy-5-methyl-4-isoxazolepropionic acid (AMPA) receptor accumulation at synapses is increased. Excitatory synaptic strength is enhanced and raises firing rates back to the set level, which represents the "homeostatic" part of the expression [46].

Metaplasticity has been described as learning-dependent changes in synaptic plasticity. So, to say, metaplasticity is a superior form of molecular plasticity mechanisms, influencing the other mechanisms.

It is also important to mention that each of these plasticity mechanism models play larger or smaller roles in different cortical areas and depend as well on developmental stages and complex, still unknown interactions.

The question of how these molecular changes exactly influence synapse-scale structural changes and how these relate to macroscopic cortical plasticity remains unanswered. It will be exciting to discover if those synaptic plasticity models, probably along with other, yet unknown mechanisms, someday can be connected to a broader principle or if there is less diverse interconnectivity then it is assumed these days.

## 6. Future prospects

So far, studies on factors that influence cortical plasticity in brachial plexus injury are scarce. Although there are multiple elegant ways of picturing structural changes on cortex in humans, such as nTMS or fMRI, without direct cortical stimulation as it is made in animal research, imaging methods are not able to reproduce plasticity on a more microscopic level. Macroscopic anatomy and rough functions of fibers can be assigned properly and molecular backgrounds of synaptic plasticity are understood to some extent as presented above. However, the connection between those two levels has to be investigated by future studies.

Another major point of interest is to understand in detail why the infant neuronal tissue has better capacities of reorganization than the adult as a basis of why, for instance, obstetric brachial plexus injuries have a better rate of recovery then the adult form. Research in this direction could someday probably benefit as a rehabilitative aspect in adult brachial plexus injury.

Generally, in the field of neurorehabilitation, not much literature can be found on aspects of rTMS rehabilitation in (surgically treated) peripheral nerve lesions. Only level A evidence was reached in the treatment of hand motor recovery in the post-acute stage of stroke, which has been investigated in rodents, as well as human subjects.

nTMS studies on the field of adult, as well as obstetric brachial plexus injuries are rare. Structured investigation in the direction of showing motor cortex plasticity sorted by diagnosis (upper brachial plexus injury, lower brachial plexus injury, isolated nerve transection) and treatment (for instance, Oberlin transfer, Leechavengvuongs transfer and so on) may help to understand cortical plasticity in brachial plexus lesions. Comparisons of nTMS with fMR images may deliver even more information.

In the future, these techniques could possibly hold the capacity of helping in decision making for timing and technique of reconstructive surgery. Also, nTMS could prospectively be helpful in prognosing the rehabilitative capacity after a peripheral nerve injury e.g. brachial plexus lesion. Preoperatively, it could be possible in the future to exactly determine the former motor area of the denervated nerve and the current motor area of the nerve donor to determine the degree of cortical plasticity that will likely happen, and thereby the chance of regaining a certain level of strength in the affected limb. It should also be easy to compare the predictive power of certain questionnaires or walking tests with the predictive power of nTMS.

All in all, nTMS seems to be a useful tool in the research of cortical plasticity after brachial plexus injury. In the best case, a study with a high number of peripheral injury patients with a surgical treatment should be created to observe cortical plasticity pre- and postoperatively and to detect more structural patterns to increase the capability of nTMS of serving as a prognostic gadget.

## 7. Conclusions

To give insight into the impact of cortical plasticity in brachial plexus injury we disentangled macroscopic and microscopic aspects. Data from human and animal studies related to cortical plasticity after peripheral nerve injury, mainly after an injury of the upper extremity, focus on timing between injury and repair. It was show that keeping a balance between waiting for spontaneous recovery and surgical repair is essential for patient outcome. The distance between the cortical areas of the donor and receptor nerve influences the time of recovery. The closer two areas are located and the better they are connected, the higher is the probability for a good outcome. A better outcome was found for rough movement in contrast to the reconstruction of fine movements, which can depend on the larger size of fine movement areas, like the hand, on motor cortex. Lowly active interneural connections probably play a larger role in cortical plasticity than it is currently understood. As they are concealed by active fibers in the healthy brain, it could be a challenge to disentangle their functions. Trauma in general is known to be a major driving force of cortical reorganization, although underlying principles still have to be fully discovered. Age strongly influences the outcome after peripheral nerve injuries. Some investigations have been made on differences in the young and adult brain concerning plasticity. Lastly, rehabilitation should already start before reconstructive surgery and should at least last two years. These were the main factors influencing outcome of a peripheral nerve injury concerning cortical plasticity. Some of them can more or less be influenced by careful planning of treatment. Reconstructive surgeons and physiotherapists should consider including this knowledge in their treatment plan.

Future research is needed to understand mechanisms of how molecular changes on a synaptic level of a neuron influence the macroscopic plasticity, to improve rehabilitative resources, to understand the exact prognostic value of nTMS in brachial plexus injury and to investigate the therapeutic capability of rTMS.

## Conflict of interest

The authors declare no conflict of interest.

## Author details

Jennifer Reinsch[1], Anna Zdunczyk[1,2], Tarik Alp Sargut[1], Maren Denker[1], Melina Engelhardt[1,2], Peter Vajkoczy[1], Thomas Picht[1,2] and Nora Dengler[1*]

1 Department of Neurosurgery, Charité Universitätsmedizin Berlin, Germany

2 Image Guidance Lab, Charité Universitätsmedizin Berlin, Germany

*Address all correspondence to: nora.dengler@charite.de

## References

[1] Ali ZS, Heuer GG, Faught RW, Kaneriya SH, Sheikh UA, Syed IS, et al. Upper brachial plexus injury in adults: comparative effectiveness of different repair techniques. J Neurosurg. 2015;122(1):195-201.

[2] Sunderland S. A classification of peripheral nerve injuries producing loss of function. Brain. 1951;74(4): 491-516.

[3] Pondaag W, van Driest FY, Groen JL, Malessy MJA. Early nerve repair in traumatic brachial plexus injuries in adults: treatment algorithm and first experiences. J Neurosurg. 2018;130(1):172-8.

[4] Songcharoen P. Management of brachial plexus injury in adults. Scand J Surg. 2008;97(4):317-23.

[5] Leechavengvongs S, Witoonchart K, Uerpairojkit C, Thuvasethakul P. Nerve transfer to deltoid muscle using the nerve to the long head of the triceps, part II: a report of 7 cases. J Hand Surg Am. 2003;28(4):633-8.

[6] Witoonchart K, Leechavengvongs S, Uerpairojkit C, Thuvasethakul P, Wongnopsuwan V. Nerve transfer to deltoid muscle using the nerve to the long head of the triceps, part I: an anatomic feasibility study. J Hand Surg Am. 2003;28(4):628-32.

[7] Foad SL, Mehlman CT, Ying J. The epidemiology of neonatal brachial plexus palsy in the United States. J Bone Joint Surg Am. 2008;90(6):1258-64.

[8] Andersen J, Watt J, Olson J, Van Aerde J. Perinatal brachial plexus palsy. Paediatr Child Health. 2006;11(2):93-100.

[9] Lombard A, Bachy M, Fitoussi F. C5-8 neonatal brachial plexus palsy. Operative findings, reconstructive strategy and outcome. J Hand Surg Eur Vol. 2020;45(8):798-804.

[10] Waters PM. Update on management of pediatric brachial plexus palsy. J Pediatr Orthop. 2005;25(1):116-26.

[11] Pondaag W, Malessy MJ. Recovery of hand function following nerve grafting and transfer in obstetric brachial plexus lesions. J Neurosurg. 2006;105(1 Suppl):33-40.

[12] Navigated Transcranial Magnetic Stimulation in Neurosurgery: Springer; 2017. 299 p.

[13] Anastakis DJ, Malessy MJ, Chen R, Davis KD, Mikulis D. Cortical plasticity following nerve transfer in the upper extremity. Hand Clin. 2008;24(4):425-44, vi-vii.

[14] Schmidt S, Bathe-Peters R, Fleischmann R, Ronnefarth M, Scholz M, Brandt SA. Nonphysiological factors in navigated TMS studies; confounding covariates and valid intracortical estimates. Hum Brain Mapp. 2015;36(1):40-9.

[15] Picht T. Current and potential utility of transcranial magnetic stimulation in the diagnostics before brain tumor surgery. CNS Oncol. 2014;3(4):299-310.

[16] Willemse RB, Hillebrand A, Ronner HE, Vandertop WP, Stam CJ. Magnetoencephalographic study of hand and foot sensorimotor organization in 325 consecutive patients evaluated for tumor or epilepsy surgery. Neuroimage Clin. 2016;10:46-53.

[17] Rossini PM, Dal Forno G. Integrated technology for evaluation of brain function and neural plasticity. Phys Med Rehabil Clin N Am. 2004;15(1):263-306.

[18] Zrenner C, Desideri D, Belardinelli P, Ziemann U. Real-time

EEG-defined excitability states determine efficacy of TMS-induced plasticity in human motor cortex. Brain Stimul. 2018;11(2):374-89.

[19] Hebb D, editor The Organization of Behavior: A Neuropsychological Theory 1949.

[20] Merzenich MM, Kaas JH, Wall J, Nelson RJ, Sur M, Felleman D. Topographic reorganization of somatosensory cortical areas 3b and 1 in adult monkeys following restricted deafferentation. Neuroscience. 1983;8(1):33-55.

[21] Jenkins WM, Merzenich MM, Recanzone G. Neocortical representational dynamics in adult primates: implications for neuropsychology. Neuropsychologia. 1990;28(6):573-84.

[22] Jacobs KM, Donoghue JP. Reshaping the cortical motor map by unmasking latent intracortical connections. Science. 1991;251(4996):944-7.

[23] Sanes JN, Suner S, Lando JF, Donoghue JP. Rapid reorganization of adult rat motor cortex somatic representation patterns after motor nerve injury. Proc Natl Acad Sci U S A. 1988;85(6):2003-7.

[24] Sanes JN, Suner S, Donoghue JP. Dynamic organization of primary motor cortex output to target muscles in adult rats. I. Long-term patterns of reorganization following motor or mixed peripheral nerve lesions. Exp Brain Res. 1990;79(3):479-91.

[25] Garraghty PE, LaChica EA, Kaas JH. Injury-induced reorganization of somatosensory cortex is accompanied by reductions in GABA staining. Somatosens Mot Res. 1991;8(4):347-54.

[26] Socolovsky M, Malessy M, Lopez D, Guedes F, Flores L. Current concepts in plasticity and nerve transfers: relationship between surgical techniques and outcomes. Neurosurg Focus. 2017;42(3):E13.

[27] Mano Y, Nakamuro T, Tamura R, Takayanagi T, Kawanishi K, Tamai S, et al. Central motor reorganization after anastomosis of the musculocutaneous and intercostal nerves following cervical root avulsion. Ann Neurol. 1995;38(1):15-20.

[28] Malessy MJ, Bakker D, Dekker AJ, Van Duk JG, Thomeer RT. Functional magnetic resonance imaging and control over the biceps muscle after intercostal-musculocutaneous nerve transfer. J Neurosurg. 2003;98(2): 261-8.

[29] Malessy MJ, van der Kamp W, Thomeer RT, van Dijk JG. Cortical excitability of the biceps muscle after intercostal-to-musculocutaneous nerve transfer. Neurosurgery. 1998;42(4):787-94; discussion 94-5.

[30] Kraus D, Naros G, Guggenberger R, Leao MT, Ziemann U, Gharabaghi A. Recruitment of Additional Corticospinal Pathways in the Human Brain with State-Dependent Paired Associative Stimulation. J Neurosci. 2018;38(6):1396-407.

[31] Gharabaghi A, Kraus D, Leao MT, Spuler M, Walter A, Bogdan M, et al. Coupling brain-machine interfaces with cortical stimulation for brain-state dependent stimulation: enhancing motor cortex excitability for neurorehabilitation. Front Hum Neurosci. 2014;8:122.

[32] Malessy MJ, Thomeer RT, van Dijk JG. Changing central nervous system control following intercostal nerve transfer. J Neurosurg. 1998;89(4):568-74.

[33] Fu SY, Gordon T. Contributing factors to poor functional recovery after delayed nerve repair: prolonged

denervation. J Neurosci. 1995;15(5 Pt 2): 3886-95.

[34] Li T, Hua XY, Zheng MX, Wang WW, Xu JG, Gu YD, et al. Different cerebral plasticity of intrinsic and extrinsic hand muscles after peripheral neurotization in a patient with brachial plexus injury: A TMS and fMRI study. Neurosci Lett. 2015;604:140-4.

[35] Simon NG, Franz CK, Gupta N, Alden T, Kliot M. Central Adaptation following Brachial Plexus Injury. World Neurosurg. 2016;85:325-32.

[36] Pondaag W, Malessy MJ. The evidence for nerve repair in obstetric brachial plexus palsy revisited. Biomed Res Int. 2014;2014:434619.

[37] Ghasemian-Shirvan E, Farnad L, Mosayebi-Samani M, Verstraelen S, Meesen RLJ, Kuo MF, et al. Age-related differences of motor cortex plasticity in adults: A transcranial direct current stimulation study. Brain Stimul. 2020;13(6):1588-99.

[38] Johnston MV. Clinical disorders of brain plasticity. Brain Dev. 2004;26(2):73-80.

[39] Fullarton AC, Myles LM, Lenihan DV, Hems TE, Glasby MA. Obstetric brachial plexus palsy: a comparison of the degree of recovery after repair of a C6 ventral root avulsion in newborn and adult sheep. Br J Plast Surg. 2001;54(8):697-704.

[40] Socolovsky M, Di Masi G, Battaglia D. Use of long autologous nerve grafts in brachial plexus reconstruction: factors that affect the outcome. Acta Neurochir (Wien). 2011;153(11):2231-40.

[41] Peter Dayan LFA. Theoretical Neuroscience: Computational and Mathematical Modeling of Neural Systems. Revised ed. Edition ed: The MIT Press; 2005. 480 p.

[42] Feldman DE, Brecht M. Map plasticity in somatosensory cortex. Science. 2005;310(5749):810-5.

[43] Fox K. Anatomical pathways and molecular mechanisms for plasticity in the barrel cortex. Neuroscience. 2002;111(4):799-814.

[44] Kim SJ, Linden DJ. Ubiquitous plasticity and memory storage. Neuron. 2007;56(4):582-92.

[45] Knott GW, Quairiaux C, Genoud C, Welker E. Formation of dendritic spines with GABAergic synapses induced by whisker stimulation in adult mice. Neuron. 2002;34(2):265-73.

[46] Turrigiano GG. The self-tuning neuron: synaptic scaling of excitatory synapses. Cell. 2008;135(3):422-35.

Section 5

# Timing

Chapter 8

# Effects of Timing of Nerve Injury and Repair in Neonatal and Adult Brachial Plexus Injury Models

*Grainne Bourke, Lev Novikov, Andrew Hart and Mikael Wiberg*

## Abstract

Brachial plexus Injury causes severe and long-term upper limb deficits at any age. The outcome from current reconstructive options depends on the severity of nerve injury and timing of intervention. This chapter summarises the differing biological responses to nerve injury that occur during neonatal, young adult and mature adult life. The central and peripheral reactions to nerve injury, the effects of timing of repair on both motor and sensory neuronal survival and basic science evidence to support early intervention are discussed.

**Keywords:** brachial plexus, nerve injury, neuronal survival

## 1. Introduction

Brachial plexus injuries (BPI) in both adults and children have serious and lifelong consequences. Fixed prognostic indicators for recovery relate to age at the time of the injury, co-morbidities and the severity and extent of the injury. Variable prognostic indictors include strategies for surgical or medical intervention and the timing of such interventions. Thus, knowledge of the best timing for intervention is critically one of the only parameters we can assess, evaluate, and optimise.

All nerve injuries, regardless of age, have both central and peripheral effects, however, these effects vary between neonates and adults. In neonates the central effects in the spinal cord after unrepaired nerve injury are early and profound with rapid cell loss while in adults the loss of motor and sensory neurons is a slower process over weeks and months and often depends on the distance from the injury site to the parent cell bodies and the type of traumatic nerve injury. Laboratory evidence to evaluate the consequences of both nerve injury and repair has demonstrated the importance in understanding the true extent of the injury including the effects over time and the benefit of early nerve repair in both adult and neonatal models.

## 2. Neonatal brachial plexus injury

Neonatal brachial plexus injury occurs at the time of birth and affects between 0.41–1.5 per 1000 live births per year. About half of these cases have a residual deficit at 6 months of age and a 25% of the cases at 12 months. Clinical examination is the current standard for assessment using either the return of elbow flexion as described by Tassin and Gilbert (1984) or the Toronto Scoring system (2002) popularised by Curtis and Clarke. Objective imaging and electrophysiological evidence to support the clinical finding is often undertaken but controversy remains about the role of these techniques in treatment decision making.

Operative exploration and reconstruction are the current gold standard in injury evaluation and intraoperative frozen sections, electrophysiology and visual nerve assessment are utilised to decide the severity of injury and the reconstructive algorithm. Even with complex peripheral nerve reconstruction these cases have long-term disability with ensuing social, psychological and economic sequelae.

### 2.1 Central effects of injury and early repair in experimental in neonatal BPI model

Retrograde degeneration of the sensory neurons in the dorsal root ganglia (DRG) and motor neurons in the spinal cord has been demonstrated in experimental neonatal brachial plexus injury models with activation of neuro inflammation and reaction of glial cells. Rapid loss of motor neurons with only 9% surviving in the anterior horn of the spinal cord at 28 days in a neonatal BPI model suggests a truly devastating reaction to nerve injury in this immature nervous system [1]. Loss of this volume of neurons so early suggests permanent long-term effects are predictable even with intervention. Timeline analysis of this early loss over 28 days post injury in one day old neonatal BPI model illustrates the loss of motor neurons apparent from day 2 after injury and continuing rapidly to fewer than 10% surviving motor neurons at 28 days from injury [1].

The methods for injury in these models have been transection and crush due to the difficulties in producing a reliable and reproducible traction model in this experimental population (weight at surgery 6–8 grammes). Clinical evidence would suggest that a traction injury would be less uniform and the possibility of associated preganglionic injury including avulsion of ventral and dorsal roots and direct spinal cord injury infers this to be an optimistic view of neuronal survival in this age group.

Other central changes to the spinal cord architecture including increased inflammatory reaction, activation of astrocytes and microglial cells and loss of synaptic boutons and dendritic branches in the anterior horn of the spinal cord.

Regarding age at the time of injury, more extensive neurological loss has been demonstrated in a sciatic nerve injury model at the age of 3–7-day old neonates when compared with 30-day old, matched neonates illustrating the fragility of the immature nervous system. In contrast to adults, distal peripheral nerve injury in neonates also results in spinal cord motor neuron loss [2, 3].

Sensory neurons are even more vulnerable to injury. Retrograde cell loss in the DRG occurs rapidly with both proximal and distal peripheral nerve injuries in neonatal experimental models [4–6].

Studies demonstrating this extensive cell death also suggest that plasticity in the spinal cord may play a role with adjacent nerve root zones compensating for the injury zone. Experiments focused on the role of C7 after unrepaired C5/C6 injury demonstrated a four -fold increase in the C7 contribution to biceps innervation [7].

Early BPI nerve repair at 1 day following injury in newborn rodents reduces the degree of retrograde motor neuron degradation with preservation of up to 20% of ventral horn motorneurons at 28 days This is a doubling of the number of preserved neurons compared with those without repair. Simultaneous decrease in activity of microglial cells and macrophages in the ventral horn supports the influence of repair on the rate and extent of neuroinflammation [1]. This has important implications for neuronal regeneration and the number of axons reaching distal targets for reinnervation.

### 2.2 Target organ changes following injury and repair in neonatal BPI model

Studies exploring the mechanism of elbow contracture in a neonatal model have highlighted the direct effects of muscle denervation on muscle tightness and the lack of fibrosis concluding that elongated sarcomeres secondary to denervation is key to elbow contracture. The underlying mechanism is likely one of increased protease activity. This mechanism of elongated denervated sarcomere length is unique to the neonatal period.

Groups with no recovery of elbow flexion had significantly more severe elbow contractures than those with even partial recovery of elbow bending. When considering the axonal counts, experimental evidence supports the inverse relationship between the number of axons and the severity of the contracture with no evidence of elbow contracture in groups that has elbow flexion motor recovery [8]. This theory can be extended to shoulder contracture but experimental modelling and the number of muscles around the shoulder girdle make this more challenging to reproduce [9].

Differential effects on fast and slow muscle fibres following denervation and reinnervation in neonatal sciatic nerve injury has also been studied by Lowrie and Vbrova [10]. In newborns both fast and slow muscle development was impaired. In contrast, they demonstrated that in slightly older (6 days of age) age groups permanent changes only occurred in fast muscle with extensive fibre loss. Slow muscle fibres suffered temporary atrophy followed by recovery once reinnervated [10].

### 2.3 Pharmacological salvage

Neuronal rescue via pharmacological manipulation has been trialled in neonatal models. P7C3, a novel class of aminopropyl carbazoles, has demonstrable influence on neuronal survival, regenerative potential of both motor and sensory neurons with ensuing end organ functional benefit. High dose N- acetylcysteine (750 mg/kg twice daily) has been shown in one neonatal study to increase motor neuronal survival in crush and transection models in this age group. There was no effect demonstrated on sensory neurons survival in this study [11].

Previous studies have also demonstrated that neurotrophic factors can provide neuroprotection for axotomised neonatal neurons following different types of nerve injury [2, 3, 6].

### 2.4 Summary and translational value

Early and rapidly progressive proximal changes in the spinal cord and DRG, combined with loss of the distal neurological architecture and the degenerative changes in the sensory and motor target organs, implies that the chance for recovery without early intervention to reinnervate the limb in global injuries seems bleak. The value of very early repair is supported by evidence that repair promotes motor neurons rescue in the anterior horn of the spinal cord. This, combined with the evidence that reinnervated muscle has the potential to adjust the elongated muscle sarcomeres associated with joint contractures in these newborn models, would encourage further translational research of the effects after early nerve repair.

Translating this experimental work to clinical practice is challenging, not only as current surgical decision making relies on clinical evaluation and recovery over a period of time but also the potential for increased anaesthetic risk in the newborn compared to the older infant. Early objective assessments that do not rely on prolonged observational recovery would be immensely helpful with this patient population. Imaging such as diffusion techniques or improved MRI that would allow earlier decision making for surgery might encourage the advent of very early surgery with the potential for preservation of motor and sensory neurons and better distal reinnervation of end organs. Previous experimental findings have shown that MRI can be used for assessment of retrograde degeneration in the dorsal root ganglia and spinal cord after peripheral nerve and spinal roots injury [12, 13].

## 3. Adult distal peripheral nerve injury

Peripheral nerve injuries to the upper limb in adults are common occurring in over 3% of trauma cases. They are more common in younger age groups and males predominate. Forearm and wrist injuries are associated with lack of full hand and upper limb functional recovery [14]. Clinical evidence supports work disability in cases of poor sensory and motor recovery. Proximal injury and type of work affect the delay in return to work [15]. Hand therapy can positively influence the outcome. Combined forearm injuries of median and ulnar nerves produce more severe deficits and as they are usually associated with injured tendons and/ or vessel injury that require more complex assessment, intervention, and rehabilitation. Most of these injuries affect the median (50%) and ulnar nerves (44%) far more frequently than the radial nerve (20%) [16]. Socioecomonic costing are considerable including care delivery, loss of income, sick days, and long-term permanent disability. Long-tern cost analysis suggests that up to 30% of patients with peripheral nerve injury have permanent disability, receiving financial compensation.

Understanding the complexity of the injury and delivering the best treatment is imperative to return to work and functional activities in this population.

Classification systems for nerve injury have been well described by Seddon and Sunderland [17, 18]. The former by way of neurapraxia, axonotmesis and neurotmesis is favoured by neurophysiologist. Neurapraxia refers to a conduction block affecting both motor and sensory nerve fibres but without Wallerian degeneration distally so the chance of functional recovery in meaningful time is high. In contrast, in axonotmesis the nerve axons and myelin sheath is injured by traction or crush but the surrounding neural sheaths are preserved. Theoretically the axons should be able to regenerate along the remaining endoneurial tubes. In neurotmesis, the axons surrounding stroma are transected or scarred, thus, unless there is intervention to overcome this gap the nerve will not recover independently. In a cohort of closed crush and traction injuries the continuity of the anatomical nerve can be difficult to confirm without surgical intervention. This suggests an overlap between these diagnostic categories.

Sunderland's classification system is more elaborate with 5 degrees of injury depending on a pathological assessment of the nerve ie. requiring histological analysis. Pathological finding ranges from myelin injury or ischaemia to axon loss and disruption of the neural sheaths surrounding the axons, fascicles or nerves. McKinnon modified this classification system to add a sixth degree describing a mixed lesion with both axon loss and conduction block occurring simultaneously within a nerve but affecting different nerve fibres [19].

Radiological assessment of nerve injury along with neurophysiological assessment in these mixed closed injuries can be challenging and surgical exploration and visualisation is often best practice.

Interventions within surgery are limited to repair, reconstruction, and repositioning of the injured nerve. Methods of nerve coaptation are varied but evidence supports simple microsurgical epineural coaptation with fascicular alignment. Historically, considerable emphasis has been placed on assessment of motor recovery as an outcome for nerve injury, repair, and reconstruction. Recent and historic papers have demonstrated that 90% of axons within peripheral nerves are afferent fibres suggesting a need to shift focus from efferent to afferent fibres to explore potential avenues of improved outcomes in nerve injury and repair [20].

### 3.1 Central effects of injury and early repair in experimental animal models

Experimental evidence has demonstrated the retrograde cell death in the dorsal root ganglion (DRG) of small diameter afferent neurons. Laboratory evidence comparing cutaneous afferent, muscular afferents and motor neurons demonstrated a greater sensitivity to injury and more profound retrograde loss in the cutaneous afferent fibres in an adult model [21, 22]. In this experimental model up to 50% of DRG neurons projecting to the mainly cutaneous sural nerve were lost after 8–24 weeks following distal sciatic nerve transection while counts of DRG neurons innervating sensory targets in the gastrocnemius muscle did not demonstrate any neuronal loss in the same timeline. Following immediate repair there was an increased survival of up to 30% of cutaneous afferent fibres with associated promotion of nerve regeneration. The significance of the distance of the injury from the cell body in influencing the extent of retrograde cell loss is important. Distal sciatic nerve injury yields sensory cell loss in the DRG over time but it does not result in detectable retrograde motor neuron loss in the anterior horn of the spinal cord in experimental mature adult animal models [22–24]. Both primary repair and peripheral nerve grafts improved the survival of sensory DRG neurons, however only about 50–60% of sensory and motor neurons regenerated into the distal nerve stump [22].

### 3.2 Target organ changes following distal nerve injury and repair

Both prolonged axotomy and prolonged denervation affect functional long-term recovery after delayed nerve repair. It is well known that nerve injury results in muscle denervation and subsequent atrophy [25]. The force and speed of muscle contraction is reduced along with a conversion to slow twitch muscle fibre type.

Degeneration of the distal nerve stump with associated Schwann cell death and fibrosis limits the nerve regeneration and subsequent recovery. Experimental work has shown that equal numbers of axons are present in the centre of nerve grafts after early (before 1 months) and late (after 3 months) reconstruction [26].

However, it is the number of axons projecting into the distal stump which decreases as time passes beyond one month after repair. Regarding the muscle fibre recovery, slow fibres predominate after denervation in the animal model gastrocnemius muscle after sciatic nerve injury and repair. This suggests they are more robust, earlier to reinnervate or preferentially reinnervated. Neuromuscular junctions are also affected by denervation. Poor reinnervation after delayed repair (greater than 3 months from injury) is supported by the presence of increased levels of embryonic specific gamma-nAChR and increased expression of MuSk (muscle specific tyrosine kinase), a coordinator of neuromuscular junction differentiation. These changes to the muscle fibre type and the neuromuscular junction in the reinnervated muscle have phenotypic consequences with changes to muscle characteristics and performance. This evidence supports the earlier repair of distal peripheral nerve injuries with better preservation of the distal stump and potential for end organ recovery.

### 3.3 Pharmacological salvage

The sensory neuronal retrograde death in the DRG following axonal injury or transection with effects on mitochondrial function and apoptosis following reactive oxygen species led to the laboratory trials of antioxidants such as N-acetylcysteine (NAC) in order to combat these changes. N acetylcysteine is a thiol containing compound that had antioxidant properties along with inhibition of proliferation and stimulation of transcriptase and enhancing intracelluar glutathione levels. Intrathecal administration of NAC combined with nerve grafting in adult distal peripheral nerve injury experimental models provides additive protective effects with increased survival (up to 90%) of DRG sensory neurons [22]. However, NAC did not affect the number of myelinated axons in the nerve graft or in the distal nerve stump, nor did it have any growth promoting effect on the spinal motoneurons in this model [22].

### 3.4 Translational implications

Nerve injuries in the forearm and hand are relatively common. Long-term cutaneous sensory deficit after nerve injury are often present at follow up assessment but recovery is often focused on recovery of the motor deficit. Perhaps this is due to the lack of sensory outcome assessment availability and the relative ease of movement evaluation. However, sensory cutaneous and muscle afferents are critical for all fluid and coordinated movements upper limb and hand movements. Loss of cutaneous sensation leads to a "blind hand" with frequent injury and accident. Earlier repair and agents such as NAC combined with focused specialist hand therapies for sensory and motor re-education may improve these outcomes in the clinical setting based on these experimental studies.

## 4. Preganglionic and postganglionic BPI in adults

Adult brachial plexus injuries occur in 1% of polytrauma cases. They are devastating life changing injuries with serious health consequences - physical, psychological, social and economic. The most common aetiology is direct collision road traffic accidents involving young male motorcyclists. Over 50% of these injuries result in complete brachial plexus injuries with permanent limb paralysis and neuropathic pain. Socioeconomic costs are high in this working population and some studies quote up to 84% partial or permanent physical disability after motorcycle accidents [27].

In this polytrauma population injuries associated with trauma brachial plexus include cervical spinal injuries, lung perforation, rib fractures, head and trunk injuries and injuries to the vasculature and bony skeleton of the upper limb and scapulothoracic association. These nerve injuries are often predominantly avulsion injuries from the spinal cord, but there remains a cohort of extraforaminal traction -rupture injuries that merit evaluation for regenerative and reconstructive potential.

Assessment of nerve injury with radiological imaging and electrophysiological investigation can be useful in identifying associated injuries that will affect prognosis, for example vascular injury or severe scapulothoracic dissociation. Improvement in MRI imaging including the advent of Diffusion Tensor Imaging to assess continuity between the spinal nerve rootlets and the spinal cord and DRG is promising. DTI also has the potential to assess nerve function and health which may provide information on the severity of nerve injury, the extent of regeneration and the recovery before the nerve reaches the sensory or motor end organ [28, 29]. Newer MRI techniques along with 3 T as opposed to 1.5 T scanning yields clearer and more defined images of the cord- rootlet junction. However even with these advanced imaging systems there are still gaps in the information acquired. Acquisition of good quality T1 images remains challenging and overall sensitivity and specificity of MRI is not 100% leaving doubt about abandoning nerve exploration when there is even the slightest possibility of nerve continuity available for reconstruction [30–34].

Clinical studies assessing the effect of presurgical delay on the outcome in upper trunk brachial plexus reconstruction in adults support a better functional outcome in cases treated within 2 months of injury. In those cases, treated later than 2 months from injury there was no significant difference in the pre and postoperative elbow flexion grade using the Medical Research Council Motor Grading System [35]. This supports relatively early surgery for brachial plexus reconstruction in adults.

### 4.1 Central effects of pre- and postganglionic plexus injury and repair

It has been demonstrated that pre- and postganglionic experimental BPI injuries in adult animals can induce significant degeneration among sensory neurons in the DRGs and motor neurons in the spinal cord [36–38].

Experimental work evaluating the neuroprotective and growth-promoting effects of early and delayed nerve grafting if the 7th cervical root has demonstrated a difference in early (4 weeks) and late (8 weeks) repair groups. In the timeline of cell loss assessment at 4 week did not demonstrate obvious sensory or motor cell loss but at 8 and 16 weeks both motor and sensory cell loss was apparent. In the anterior horn the motor loss increased from 15–29% between 8 and 16 weeks and in the DRG the sensory neuron loss increased from 32–50%. Both early repair and delayed repair were effective in preventing retrograde degeneration of motoneurons but of course the repairs at 8 weeks have far fewer neurons remaining in any case [37]. Neither early nor late repair were able to rescue sensory neurons but again the population was higher in the early repair group. In both groups the proportion of regenerating neurons remained constant. Thus, although delayed nerve repair is neuroprotective it will only protect those remaining neurons. This evidence supports the proposal that early nerve repair is optimal to promote best motor and sensory recovery and even this is at considerable loss of both motor and sensory neurons. Avulsion of the ventral root in the adult lumbar cord yields 40–80% neuronal cell death at 2–4 weeks from injury [39–41]. This, combined with the technical difficulties of any type of root reimplantation due to the disruption to normal architecture, have forced the field of reconstruction surgery after avulsion injury nearer the end organ in nerve transfers from adjacent functioning motor or sensory nerves.

Experimental evaluation of primary and secondary changes visible on MRI imaging of the spinal ventral root after transection and avulsion of a lumbar plexus model has also been completed [12]. MRI and histological analysis of the ventral horn demonstrated differences in the volume of the ventral horn on MRI with avulsion injury which is not apparent with transection injury. Histological analysis of these imaged ventral horns revealed severe loss of neurons, dendrites, axons, and synapses with increases in microglial cells and astrocytes. It is suggested that the loss of neuronal cells may contribute to the change in MRI signal leading to the changes in the images acquired.

### 4.2 Pharmacological intervention and salvage

Experimental evidence exists that supports that the use of NAC can prevent active death after proximal sensory nerve injury [42]. Suggested pathways include mitochondrial pathway blockade to inhibit caspase cascade. In ventral horn motor neurons NAC is also protective (>90%) with dose dependent effects. In avulsion injuries the response to NAC was diluted to 70% suggesting the immediate necrosis of neuronal cells at the time of injury to be a significant factor in cell loss. Regarding delivery methods intrathecal was more effective than intraperitoneal but the later is more practical and clinically relevant suggesting systemic therapy would be effective. Such therapies are already used for acetaminophen overdose and toxicity [43]. Timing of intervention is important considering the very early and rapid loss of both sensory and slightly less rapid loss of motor neurons with proximal transection or avulsion injuries. In addition, earlier studies also demonstrated the efficacy of prolonged intrathecal treatment with various neurotrophic factors to prevent retrograde cells death in both the DRGs and spinal cord [40, 44]. However, significant side effect on the rate of axon regeneration and normal synaptic composition could significantly limit their potential clinical application [41, 45].

## 5. Summary

Central and peripheral effects of nerve injuries in neonates, young adults and mature adults have been studied experimentally. Loss of neurons is seen in all age groups, but early rapid loss is particularly apparent in neonates and in sensory neurons in all age groups. Early repair has neuroprotective properties, but cell loss is still significant even with almost immediate intervention. These experimental studies support nerve repair as soon as is safely possible given the other associated injuries in both adult and neonatal populations. Proximal nerve injuries such as brachial plexus injuries are particularly damaging to the motor and sensory nerve pool. Avulsion injuries in adults have similar devastating levels of neuronal cell loss when compared with neonatal transection injuries. However, early repair is technically very challenging is avulsion injuries due to the associated necrosis of the supporting ventral horn cell architecture. Pharmacological antioxidant therapies have been neuroprotective in adult studies and may be particularly relevant to sensory neuronal support.


## Author details

Grainne Bourke[1,2,3]*, Lev Novikov[3], Andrew Hart[3] and Mikael Wiberg[3]

1 Department of Plastic and Reconstructive Surgery, Leeds Teaching Hospitals Trust, Leeds, UK

2 Leeds Institute for Medical Research, University of Leeds, Leeds, UK

3 Department of Integrative Medical Biology, University of Umea, Sweden

*Address all correspondence to: grainnebourke@nhs.net

## References

[1] Bourke, G., McGrath, A. M., Wiberg, M., & Novikov, L. N. (2018). Effects of early nerve repair on experimental brachial plexus injury in neonatal rats. J Hand Surg Eur *43*(3), 275-281. doi:10.1177/1753193417732696

[2] Vejsada, R., Sagot, Y., & Kato, A. C. (1995). Quantitative comparison of the transient rescue effects of neurotrophic factors on axotomized motoneurons in vivo. Eur J Neurosci, *7*(1), 108-115. doi:10.1111/j.1460-9568.1995.tb01025.x

[3] Vejsada, R., Tseng, J. L., Lindsay, R. M., Acheson, A., Aebischer, P., & Kato, A. C. (1998). Synergistic but transient rescue effects of BDNF and GDNF on axotomized neonatal motoneurons. Neuroscience, *84*(1), 129-139. doi:10.1016/s0306-4522(97)00497-1

[4] Himes, B. T., & Tessler, A. (1989). Death of some dorsal root ganglion neurons and plasticity of others following sciatic nerve section in adult and neonatal rats. J Comp Neurol, *284*(2), 215-230. doi:10.1002/cne.902840206

[5] Lowrie, M. B., & Vrbova, G. (1992). Dependence of postnatal motoneurones on their targets: review and hypothesis. Trends Neurosci, *15*(3), 80-84. doi:10.1016/0166-2236(92)90014-y

[6] Snider, W. D., Elliott, J. L., & Yan, Q. (1992). Axotomy-induced neuronal death during development. J Neurobiol, 23(9), 1231-1246. doi:10.1002/neu.480230913

[7] Korak, K. J., Tam, S. L., Gordon, T., Frey, M., & Aszmann, O. C. (2004). Changes in spinal cord architecture after brachial plexus injury in the newborn. Brain, *127*(Pt 7), 1488-1495. doi:10.1093/brain/awh155

[8] Weekley, H., Nikolaou, S., Hu, L., Eismann, E., Wylie, C., & Cornwall, R. (2012). The effects of denervation, reinnervation, and muscle imbalance on functional muscle length and elbow flexion contracture following neonatal brachial plexus injury. J Orthop Res, *30*(8), 1335-1342. doi:10.1002/jor.22061

[9] Nikolaou, S., Cramer, A. A., Hu, L., Goh, Q., Millay, D. P., & Cornwall, R. (2019). Proteasome inhibition preserves longitudinal growth of denervated muscle and prevents neonatal neuromuscular contractures. JCI Insight, *4*(23). doi:10.1172/jci.insight.128454

[10] Lowrie, M. B., & Vrbova, G. (1984). Different pattern of recovery of fast and slow muscles following nerve injury in the rat. J Physiol, *349*, 397-410. doi:10.1113/jphysiol.1984.sp015163

[11] Catapano, J., Zhang, J., Scholl, D., Chiang, C., Gordon, T., & Borschel, G. H. (2017). N-Acetylcysteine Prevents Retrograde Motor Neuron Death after Neonatal Peripheral Nerve Injury. Plast Reconstr Surg 139(5), 1105e-1115e. doi:10.1097/PRS.0000000000003257

[12] Karalija, A., Novikova, L. N., Oradd, G., Wiberg, M., & Novikov, L. N. (2016). Differentiation of Pre- and Postganglionic Nerve Injury Using MRI of the Spinal Cord. PLoS One, *11*(12), e0168807. doi:10.1371/journal.pone.0168807

[13] West, C. A., Davies, K. A., Hart, A. M., Wiberg, M., Williams, S. R., & Terenghi, G. (2007). Volumetric magnetic resonance imaging of dorsal root ganglia for the objective quantitative assessment of neuron death after peripheral nerve injury. Exp Neurol, *203*(1), 22-33. doi:10.1016/j.expneurol.2006.07.013

[14] Padovano, W. M., Dengler, J., Patterson, M. M., Yee, A., Snyder-Warwick, A. K., Wood, M. D.,

Mackinnon, S. E. (2020). Incidence of Nerve Injury After Extremity Trauma in the United States. Hand (N Y), 1558944720963895. doi:10.1177/1558944720963895

[15] Jaquet, J. B., Luijsterburg, A. J., Kalmijn, S., Kuypers, P. D., Hofman, A., & Hovius, S. E. (2001). Median, ulnar, and combined median-ulnar nerve injuries: functional outcome and return to productivity. J Trauma, *51*(4), 687-692. doi:10.1097/00005373-200110000-00011

[16] Bergmeister, K. D., Grosse-Hartlage, L., Daeschler, S. C., Rhodius, P., Bocker, A., Beyersdorff, M., Harhaus, L. (2020). Acute and long-term costs of 268 peripheral nerve injuries in the upper extremity. PLoS One, *15*(4), e0229530. doi:10.1371/journal.pone.0229530

[17] Seddon, R. J. (1947). Surgical experiences with peripheral nerve injuries. Q Bull Northwest Univ Med Sch, 21(3), 201-210. https://www.ncbi.nlm.nih.gov/pubmed/20255894

[18] Sunderland, S. (1951). A classification of peripheral nerve injuries producing loss of function. Brain, 74(4), 491-516. doi:10.1093/brain/74.4.491

[19] Robinson, L. R. (2000). Traumatic injury to peripheral nerves. Muscle Nerve, *23*(6), 863-873. doi:10.1002/(sici)1097-4598(200006)23:6<863::aid-mus4>3.0.co;2-0

[20] Gesslbauer, B., Hruby, L. A., Roche, A. D., Farina, D., Blumer, R., & Aszmann, O. C. (2017). Axonal components of nerves innervating the human arm. Ann Neurol, *82*(3), 396-408. doi:10.1002/ana.25018

[21] Hu, P., & McLachlan, E. M. (2003). Selective reactions of cutaneous and muscle afferent neurons to peripheral nerve transection in rats. J Neurosci *23*(33), 10559-10567. https://www.ncbi.nlm.nih.gov/pubmed/14627640

[22] Welin, D., Novikova, L. N., Wiberg, M., Kellerth, J. O., & Novikov, L. N. (2008). Survival and regeneration of cutaneous and muscular afferent neurons after peripheral nerve injury in adult rats. Exp Brain Res, *186*(2), 315-323. doi:10.1007/s00221-007-1232-5

[23] McKay Hart, A., Brannstrom, T., Wiberg, M., & Terenghi, G. (2002). Primary sensory neurons and satellite cells after peripheral axotomy in the adult rat: timecourse of cell death and elimination. Exp Brain Res, *142*(3), 308-318. doi:10.1007/s00221-001-0929-0

[24] Tandrup, T., Woolf, C. J., & Coggeshall, R. E. (2000). Delayed loss of small dorsal root ganglion cells after transection of the rat sciatic nerve. J Comp Neurol, *422*(2), 172-180. doi:10.1002/(sici)1096-9861(20000626)422:2<172::aid-cne2>3.0.co;2-h

[25] Wong, A., & Pomerantz, J. H. (2019). The Role of Muscle Stem Cells in Regeneration and Recovery after Denervation: A Review. Plast Reconstr Surg, *143*(3), 779-788. doi:10.1097/PRS.0000000000005370

[26] Jonsson, S., Wiberg, R., McGrath, A. M., Novikov, L. N., Wiberg, M., Novikova, L. N., & Kingham, P. J. (2013). Effect of delayed peripheral nerve repair on nerve regeneration, Schwann cell function and target muscle recovery. PLoS One, *8*(2), e56484. doi:10.1371/journal.pone.0056484

[27] Bittar, C. K., Cliquet, A., Costa, V., Pacheco, A. C. F., & Ricci, R. L. (2020). Socioeconomic Impact of Motorcycle Accident Victims in the Emergency Room of a Hospital (Part 2). Acta Ortop Bras, *28*(3), 149-151. doi:10.1590/1413-785220202803230036

[28] Wade, R. G., Teh, I., Andersson, G., Yeh, F. C., Wiberg, M., & Bourke, G. (2021). Fractional anisotropy thresholding for deterministic

tractography of the roots of the brachial plexus. Sci Rep, *11*(1), 80. doi:10.1038/s41598-020-79840-8

[29] Wade, R. G., Whittam, A., Teh, I., Andersson, G., Yeh, F. C., Wiberg, M., & Bourke, G. (2020c). Diffusion tensor imaging of the roots of the brachial plexus: a systematic review and meta-analysis of normative values. Clin Transl Imaging, *8*(6), 419-431. doi:10.1007/s40336-020-00393-x

[30] Wade, R. G., Bligh, E. R., Nar, K., Stone, R. S., Roberts, D. J., Teh, I., & Bourke, G. (2020a). The Geometry of the roots of the Brachial Plexus. J Anat, *237*(6), 999-1005. doi:10.1111/joa.13270

[31] Wade, R. G., Itte, V., Rankine, J. J., Ridgway, J. P., & Bourke, G. (2018a). The diagnostic accuracy of 1.5T magnetic resonance imaging for detecting root avulsions in traumatic adult brachial plexus injuries. J Hand Surg Eur Vol, *43*(3), 250-258. doi:10.1177/1753193417729587

[32] Wade, R. G., Takwoingi, Y., Wormald, J. C. R., Ridgway, J. P., Tanner, S., Rankine, J. J., & Bourke, G. (2018b). Magnetic resonance imaging for detecting root avulsions in traumatic adult brachial plexus injuries: protocol for a systematic review of diagnostic accuracy. Syst Rev, *7*(1), 76. doi:10.1186/s13643-018-0737-2

[33] Wade, R. G., Takwoingi, Y., Wormald, J. C. R., Ridgway, J. P., Tanner, S., Rankine, J. J., & Bourke, G. (2019). MRI for Detecting Root Avulsions in Traumatic Adult Brachial Plexus Injuries: A Systematic Review and Meta-Analysis of Diagnostic Accuracy. Radiology, *293*(1), 125-133. doi:10.1148/radiol.2019190218

[34] Wade, R. G., Tanner, S. F., Teh, I., Ridgway, J. P., Shelley, D., Chaka, B., Bourke, G. (2020b). Diffusion Tensor Imaging for Diagnosing Root Avulsions in Traumatic Adult Brachial Plexus Injuries: A Proof-of-Concept Study. Front Surg, *7*, 19. doi:10.3389/fsurg.2020.00019

[35] Jivan, S., Kumar, N., Wiberg, M., & Kay, S. (2009). The influence of pre-surgical delay on functional outcome after reconstruction of brachial plexus injuries. J Plast Reconstr Aesthet Surg, *62*(4), 472-479. doi:10.1016/j.bjps.2007.11.027

[36] Gu, Y., Spasic, Z., & Wu, W. (1997). The effects of remaining axons on motoneuron survival and NOS expression following axotomy in the adult rat. Dev Neurosci, *19*(3), 255-259. doi:10.1159/000111214

[37] Jivan, S., Novikova, L. N., Wiberg, M., & Novikov, L. N. (2006). The effects of delayed nerve repair on neuronal survival and axonal regeneration after seventh cervical spinal nerve axotomy in adult rats. Exp Brain Res, *170*(2), 245-254. doi:10.1007/s00221-005-0207-7

[38] Ma, J., Novikov, L. N., Wiberg, M., & Kellerth, J. O. (2001). Delayed loss of spinal motoneurons after peripheral nerve injury in adult rats: a quantitative morphological study. Exp Brain Res, *139*(2), 216-223. doi:10.1007/s002210100769

[39] Koliatsos, V. E., Price, W. L., Pardo, C. A., & Price, D. L. (1994). Ventral root avulsion: an experimental model of death of adult motor neurons. J Comp Neurol, *342*(1), 35-44. doi:10.1002/cne.903420105

[40] Novikov, L., Novikova, L., & Kellerth, J. O. (1997). Brain-derived neurotrophic factor promotes axonal regeneration and long-term survival of adult rat spinal motoneurons in vivo. Neuroscience, *79*(3), 765-774. doi:10.1016/s0306-4522(96)00665-3

[41] Novikov, L. N., Novikova, L. N., Holmberg, P., & Kellerth, J. (2000).

Exogenous brain-derived neurotrophic factor regulates the synaptic composition of axonally lesioned and normal adult rat motoneurons. Neuroscience, *100*(1), 171-181. doi:10.1016/s0306-4522(00)00256-6

[42] Zhang, C. G., Welin, D., Novikov, L., Kellerth, J. O., Wiberg, M., & Hart, A. M. (2005). Motorneuron protection by N-acetyl-cysteine after ventral root avulsion and ventral rhizotomy. Br J Plast Surg, *58*(6), 765-773. doi:10.1016/j.bjps.2005.04.012

[43] Chiew, A. L., Gluud, C., Brok, J., & Buckley, N. A. (2018). Interventions for paracetamol (acetaminophen) overdose. Cochrane Database Syst Rev, *2*, CD003328. doi:10.1002/14651858.CD003328.pub3

[44] Ljungberg, C., Novikov, L., Kellerth, J. O., Ebendal, T., & Wiberg, M. (1999). The neurotrophins NGF and NT-3 reduce sensory neuronal loss in adult rat after peripheral nerve lesion. Neurosci Lett, *262*(1), 29-32. doi:10.1016/s0304-3940(99)00040-3

[45] Gold, B. G. (1997). Axonal regeneration of sensory nerves is delayed by continuous intrathecal infusion of nerve growth factor. Neuroscience, *76*(4), 1153-1158. doi:10.1016/s0306-4522(96)00416-2

## Section 6

# New Ways of Thinking

Chapter 9

# A Funhouse Mirror: Muscular Co-Contractions as a Reflection of a Spontaneous Aberrant Regeneration of the Brachial Plexus Injury in the Adults - Anatomical Background, an Attempt to Classify and Their Clinical Relevance within the Reconstruction Strategies

*Alexander A. Gatskiy and Ihor B. Tretyak*


## Abstract

A certain number of spontaneously recovering birth injuries to the brachial (BPI) plexus are known to be accompanied by muscle co-contractions (Co-Cs). The process of aberrant spontaneous regeneration contributes to the appearance of this phenomenon. Treatment strategies are mostly narrowed down to temporarily "switching off" the antagonist, allowing the agonist to perform. Less is known about the incidence of BPI-associated Co-Cs in adults (a-BPI), the control of which mainly presumes the extrapolation of a treatment strategy that has been shown to be effective in infants. Nowadays, surgical reconstruction of independent elbow flexion at BPIs relies heavily on redirection (transfer) of nerves that produce their own Co-Cs. These induced Co-Cs could potentially be reduced. Selecting the appropriate nerve transfer strategy (when the donor pool is narrowing), with its potential impact on the already complex and intricate global and segmental biomechanics of the upper extremity, becomes challenging. The chapter presents the anatomical background for the occurrence of muscular Co-Cs, a work on clinical classification of both regeneration associated and induced Co-Cs, possible surgical strategies, their benefits and limitations, in the presence of regeneration-associated muscle Co-Cs at a-BPI and clinical examples.


**Keywords:** adult brachial plexus injury, nerve transfer, medial pectoral nerve, oberlin transfer, musculocutaneous nerve, co-contraction

## 1. Introduction

Brachial plexus injury (BPI) in adults (a-BPI) remains one of the leading causes of permanent and severe disability among all injuries in the peripheral nervous system [1]. The evolution of treatment options from neurolysis through nerve grafting to nerve transfers has led to dramatic improvements in functional outcomes [2]. The timing of the surgical reconstruction has always been strongly dependent on the process of spontaneous regeneration [3]. As the time allotted for spontaneous regeneration passes and no clear clinical and electrophysiological signs of regeneration are seen, the majority of surgeons advocate for active surgical reconstruction [4].

The dynamics of spontaneous regeneration are well described in newborns with obstetric BPI [4, 5]. It is often accompanied by co-contractions (Co-C) of *de novo* reinnervated muscles [6], which respond well to injections of botulinum toxin A [7]. Less information can be found concerning the management of the Co-C in cases of a-BPI [8].

A rational explanation of the origin of the Co-Cs could be a change in the predominance of root representation within the muscles of the upper extremity in the case of BPI (**Figure 1**). This predominance is present both under normal conditions (known as "luxury innervation" [9]) and becomes more evident under the described [10, 11] pathological conditions (known as injury/regeneration associated "simple and complex misdirection"). For instance, at nonfunctioning C5-C6 rootlets greater pectoral, triceps brachii, latissimus dorsi muscles, etc. receive motor fascicles from C7-8-Th1, thus, have or receive closely adjoined motor cortex representation. The activation of the closely adjoined motor cortex during voluntary contraction could possibly lead to their co-activation Co-C. The clinically apparent expression of Co-C most probably depends on how close the cortical centers are situated. Functional MRI (cortical mapping) findings partially explain this process [12].

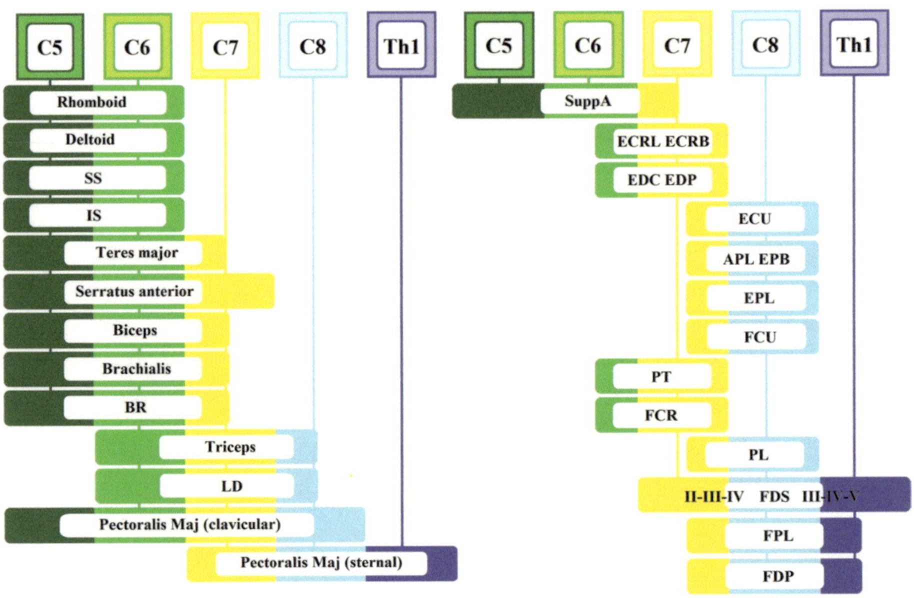


**Figure 1.**
*Normal representation of the roots' of the brachial plexus within the muscles of the upper extremity (a similar color represents the same innervation pattern or representation of roots in the muscles and is most likely responsible for the occurrence of co-contraction(s)). SS—suprascapular muscle; IS—infrascapular muscle; BR—brachioradialis; LD—latissimus dorsi muscle; SuppA—supinator antebrachii muscle; ECRL—extensor carpi radialis longus; ECRB—extensor carpi radialis brevis; EDC—extensor digitorum communis; EDP—extensor indicis and digiti minimi; ECU—extensor carpi ulnaris; APL—abductor pollicis brevis; EPB—extensor pollicis brevis; EPL—extensor pollicis longus; FCU—flexor carpi ulnaris; PT—pronator teres muscle; FDS—flexor digitorum superficilalis; FPL—flexor pollicis longus; FDP—flexor digitorum profundus.*

## 2. From clinical observations to systematic approach to classification: what we know exactly

To date, there is no classification of muscular Co-Cs of the upper extremity associated with *"aberrant spontaneous"* BPI recovery. Later descriptions of this pathologic motor phenomenon are narrowed to so-called "triceps syndrome" [13], which includes co-activation of both biceps and triceps brachii muscles *"antagonistic"* Co-C (**Table 1**). However, other types of co-activation have not received much attention, regardless of the fact that they potentially could severely entangle the biomechanics of the proximal and distal segments of the upper extremity. The clinically observed *"proximal-proximal"* Co-C (**Table 1**) related to "triceps syndrome" includes also simultaneous activation of the triceps brachii and greater pectoral muscle *"non-antagonistic"* (**Table 1**). Even less is known about the distal projection of "triceps syndrome" on the functions of the wrist and fingers. The clinical observations that have already been made have not yet been reflected in any type of scientific literature. Still, elbow, wrist, and finger extension, or *"proximal-distal"* Co-C (**Table 1**) is not uncommon. Technically, this type of co-activation is not a pure Co-C, hence the wrist and finger extension does not occur simultaneously, but rather sequentially in relation to the contraction of the triceps brachii muscle. Yet it is still present within the clinical picture of "triceps syndrome" and dramatically entangles wrist/hand function and stability.

Currently, injuries to BPI are mainly treated with nerve transfers (NT) [14]. The pool of traditional extra- and intraplexal donor nerves could be narrowed due to cranially (involvement of C4) and/or caudally expanded (involvement of C7-8) BPI, respectively. In most cases, it consists of Oberlin [15], double-fascicular [16], and medial pectoral [12] NTs.

It is well known that any type of NT, especially when a donor-nerve provides motor fascicles to more than a single muscle, could potentially produce co-activation (*"induced"* Co-C **Table 1**) of other muscles related to the donor's nerve during the early stages of clinically visible regeneration [17]. Reduction of this type of co-activation is achieved through active rehabilitation programs [17]. Most of the programs are aimed at dissociating the voluntary activation of the newly obtained function from the entire area of the cortical representation of the donor nerve [17]. The widespread adoption of NTs among the surgical society quickly isolated a pool of unwanted NTs. These NTs were able to produce induced Co-C [18] and were mostly related to the

| **Aberrant spontaneous** | | **Induced** | |
|---|---|---|---|
| **Proximal-Proximal** | *Example: BB-TB-Pct* | **Proximal-Proximal** | *Example (nerves): Pct-BB (PM-MCN)* |
| Proximal-Distal* | *Example: TB-ECRB/L* | Proximal-Distal | *Example (nerves): FCU/FDP4–5-BB (UN-MCN)* |
| Distal-Distal* | *Example: WE-FE* | Distal-Distal | *Example (Nerves): FCR-EDC (MN-PIN)* |
| Antagonistic | *Example: BB-TB* | Extraplexal | *Example (nerves): Diaphr.-BB (PhN-MCN)* |
| Non-antagonistic | *Example: TB-Pct* | Intraplexal | *Example (nerves): any known* |
| Only intraplexal | *Example: any known* | Antagonism** | *Example**:?* |

*BB—biceps brachii muscle; Pct—greater pectoral muscle; TB—triceps brachii muscle; ECRB/L—extensor carpi radialis brevis et longus; WE—wrist extensors; FE—finger extensors; FCU—flexor carpi ulnaris; FPD4–5—deep flexors of 4–5 fingers; EDC—extensor digitorum communis; Diaphr.—diaphragm; PM—pectoral nerves; MCN—musculocutaneous nerve; UN—ulnar nerve; MN—median nerve; PIN—posterior interosseous nerve.*
**Sequential Co-C (see description in the text)*
***Unknown.*

**Table 1.**
*Work classification of known Co-Cs.*

forearm (*"distal-distal"* Co-C **Table 1**). In most cases, attempts to dissociate them were unsuccessful and severely confounded the hand-wrist biomechanics [18].

Reconstructions strategies in BPI are prioritizing the reanimation of the elbow flexion [3, 19]. Active surgical reconstruction, with both tendon and NTs, provides active elbow flexion in either earlier or later terms [8]. The general principles of NTs are well known [20]. Reconstruction strategies of BPI are strongly dependent on the selection of an appropriate donor nerve, considering the possible functional advantages and disadvantages of each.

Hence, the evaluation of the efficacy of any type of NT is generally narrowed to the identification of either a muscular power (MRC) or a change in a joint angle produced by the recovered muscle, Oberlin or double-fascicular NT have become most popular and have established themselves as a "golden standard" [2]. The induced *"proximal-distal"* (**Table 1**) Co-C, which follows the abovementioned procedures, is one of those that are easily nullified even without any extensive reeducation [17].

On the other hand, the influence of a nerve transfer on the intimate biomechanical correlation between the upper arm and hand movements is underestimated in most cases. Only a few publications have attempted to characterize and define the real meaning of this coordination and the influence of induced proximal-distal co-activation on the affected limb on a global scale [17]. Escudero et al. [17] discovered that at least 39% of patients who received Oberlin transfer were unable to dissociate elbow flexion from wrist/finger flexion. From a biomechanical point of view, this meant that it deeply "confounded" the function of the hand during daily activities [17].

The interaction between aberrant and induced Co-C in the case of BPI, its influence on the global biomechanics of the upper extremity has not received any reflection in the scientific literature at all. This is most likely due to its extremely rare occurrence among all cases of a BPI. Moreover, since the use of reconstructive strategies presumes the return of lost functions and the preservation (or at least not the loss of the majority) of the preserved ones, the following clinical examples could potentially be of great interest.

## 3. Clinical examples

### 3.1 Clinical example 1

A 26-year-old man was admitted to our department 2 mos. after a traction-type injury to his right brachial plexus in a motorcycle accident; neurological examination revealed complete injury to the right brachial plexus. A C5-6-7-8 avulsion with no cranial expansion and preserved function to n.phrenicus (C4) was confirmed during the explorative surgery. None of the intra-plexal motor donor nerves were available for transfer at the time of surgery. In order to reanimate active elbow flexion, NT of n.phrenicus to the musculocutaneous nerve (distally to the branches of the coracobrachialis muscle) through approx. 12 cm sural nerve graft was performed. Another NT of the accessory to the suprascapular nerve [21] was performed to reanimate abduction and external rotation of the shoulder.

Physiotherapy was resumed 6 weeks later. 13 mos. after surgery, shoulder abduction (frontal plane) and external rotation were 80° and 40°, respectively. BB recovered to M4 and elbow flexion was near 90°, was associated with breathing "breathing hand" *induced Co-C.* Voluntary elbow flexion appeared on the 16th mo. and could be controlled consciously. 19 mos. after the surgery, we observed the recovery to the function of the greater pectoral muscle (M4), which was associated with ineffective (less than M2) function to FDPs - *aberrant spontaneous proximal-distal Co-C (Pct-FF)* (**Figure 2**). A T-shaped wrist plate and trapeziometacarpal

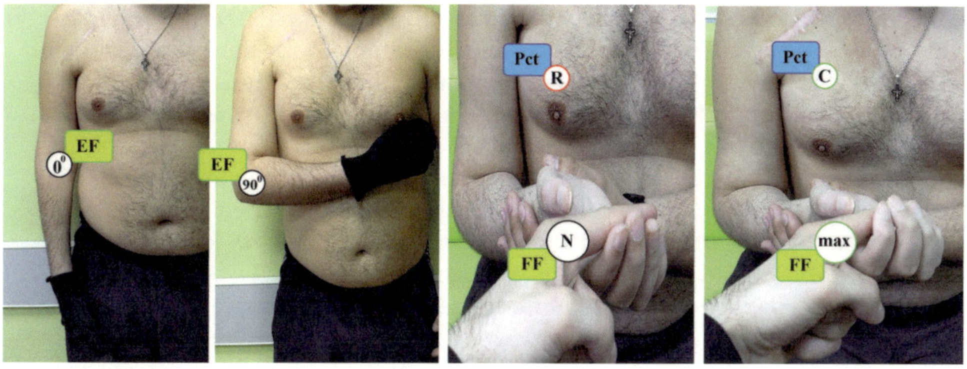


**Figure 2.**
*"Breathing hand" andcorrelation between greater pectoral muscle function and finger flexion (late proximal-distal Co-C). EF—elbow flexion; Pct—greater pectoral muscle, FF—finger flexion; N—neutral position; R—rest; C—maximal contraction; max—maximal finger flexion/transverse volar grip.*

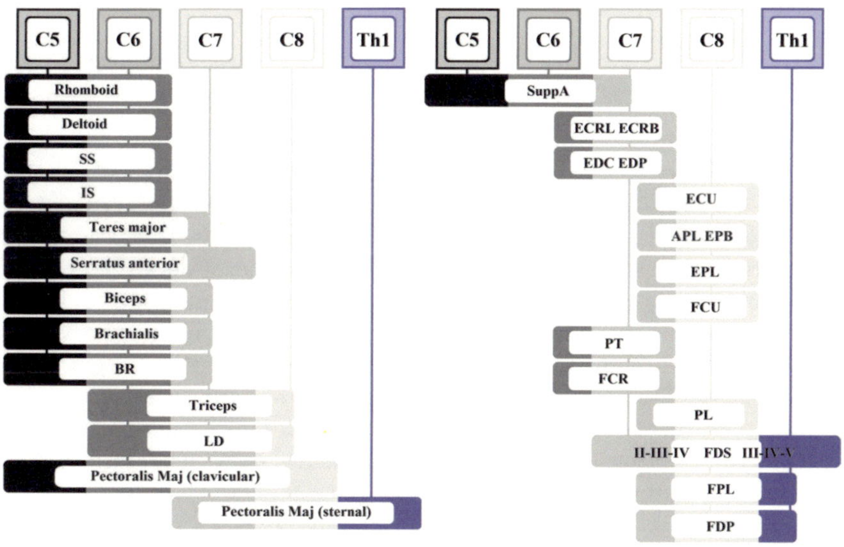


**Figure 3.**
*Schematic explanation of the occurrence of late proximal-distal Co-C (Pct-FF) associated with aberrant spontaneous regeneration of initially complete a-BPI (a similar color represents the same innervation pattern or representation of roots within muscles and is most likely responsible for the emergence of co-contraction). SS—suprascapular muscle; IS—infrascapular muscle; BR—brachioradialis; LD—latissimus dorsi muscle; SuppA—supinator antebrachii muscle; ECRL—extensor carpi radialis longus; ECRB—extensor carpi radialis brevis; EDC—extensor digitorum communis; EDP—extensor indicis and digiti minimi; ECU—extensor carpi ulnaris; APL—abductor pollicis brevis; EPB—extensor pollicis brevis; EPL—extensor pollicis longus; FCU—flexor carpi ulnaris; PT—pronator teres muscle; FDS—flexor digitorum superficilalis; FPL—flexor pollicis longus; FDP—flexor digitorum profundus.*

arthrodesis were performed to ensure the stability of the hand, and active rehabilitation started 4 weeks after the surgery. The patient was instructed to navigate the finger flexion by actively contracting the greater pectoral muscle with maximum effort. 24 mos. after the initial surgery, the FDP power increased to M3–4, allowing the patient to perform an effective transverse volar grip.

*Rational explanation:* It is not uncommon for some muscle groups to regenerate to a certain degree in many later terms after complete injury to the brachial plexus. Most often, regeneration in the case of complete a-BPI occurs in a greater pectoral muscle. Acting as an internal rotator of the shoulder, its function disables "sagittalization" of the upper arm and forearm during the basic activities of daily living

(ADLs), especially when external rotators are non-functional or regenerated to a much lesser extent in terms of power. The shortening of the muscle and tendon structures surrounding the glenohumeral joint confirms this functional misposition. Only a small number of complete a-BPIs show muscle regeneration on any surface of the forearm, even rarely to hand intrinsics. It is a common occurrence, and this clinical example confirms that late spontaneous regeneration of both the greater pectoral and forearm muscles is accompanied by their co-activation. Technically, this type of co-activation does comply with the previously classified subtypes (**Table 1**) and comprises the characteristics of "*proximal-distal non-antagonistic Co-C*". The explanation for the occurrence of this late Co-C lies most probably within the innervation pattern of the aforementioned muscles (**Figure 3**).

*Conclusion:* The recovered function of the greater pectoral muscle serves as an indicator of a likelihood of recovery of other distal muscles (forearm) of the upper extremity, playing a leading role in a co-activation pair in this particular case the greater pectoral muscle helped to navigate the contraction of the FDPs, providing not only clinically visible feedback but also an EMG-assisted video-feedback during active rehabilitation.

### 3.2 Clinical example 2

A 28-year-old man was admitted to our department 3 mos. after a traction-type injury to the left brachial plexus in a motorcycle accident; neurological examination revealed the complete injury to the left brachial plexus. A C5-6 avulsion with no cranial expansion and preserved function to n.phrenicus (C4) was confirmed during the explorative surgery. None of the intraplexal motor donor nerves were available for transfer at the time of surgery. In order to reanimate active elbow flexion, NT of n.phrenicus was transferred to the musculocutaneous nerve (distally to the branches of the coracobrachialis muscle) through a sural nerve graft approximately 12 cm long. Two other NTs were performed to reanimate flexion, abduction, and external rotation of the shoulder: pars sternocleidomastoideus of the accessory nerve to the axillary nerve through approx. 14 cm sural nerve graft and suprascapular nerve [21] NT, respectively.

Physiotherapy was resumed 6 weeks later. 17 mos. after surgery, shoulder abduction (frontal plane) was 90°. BB recovered to M4, and elbow flexion was near 110°, was associated with breathing—the "breathing hand" *induced Co-C*. Voluntary elbow flexion could be controlled consciously 24 mos. after surgery, we observed the recovery of function of the greater pectoral muscle (M4), which was associated with the effective (M4) function of ECRB—*aberrant spontaneous proximal-distal Co-C (Pct-WE)* (**Figure 4**). A T-shaped wrist plate and a trapeziometacarpal arthrodesis were performed to ensure wrist stability, followed by a rigid cast

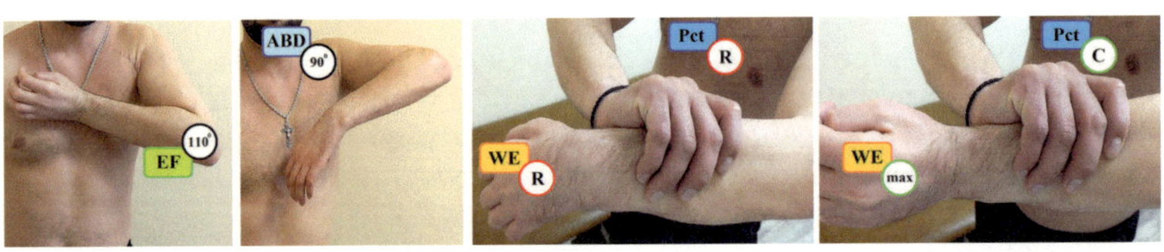


**Figure 4.**
*"Breathing hand", shoulder abduction and correlation between greater pectoral muscle function and wrist extension (late proximal-distal* Co-C before wrist arthrodesis). EF—elbow flexion; ABD—shoulder abduction; Pct—greater pectoral muscle, WE—wrist extension; R—rest; C—maximal contraction; max—maximal wrist extension mediated by ECRB.*

immobilization for the next 2 mos. Recovered function to ECRB associated with late *aberrant spontaneous proximal-distal Co-C (Pct-WE)* will be used for a tendon transfer to restore FDP/FPL function at a later date.

*Rational explanation:* It is not uncommon for some muscle groups to regenerate to a certain degree at a later date after complete injury to the brachial plexus. Most often, regeneration at complete a-BPI occurs in the greater pectoral muscle. Acting as an internal rotator of the shoulder, its function disables "sagittalization" of the upper arm and forearm during basic activities of daily living (ADLs), especially when external rotators are non-functional or are regenerated to a much lesser extent in terms of power. The shortening of the muscle and tendon structures surrounding the glenohumeral joint confirms this functional mis-position. Only a small number of complete a-BPIs show muscle regeneration of either surface of the forearm, even rarely to hand intrinsics. This is a common occurrence, and this clinical example confirms that late spontaneous regeneration of both the greater pectoral and forearm muscles is accompanied by their co-activation. Technically, this type of co-activation does comply with previously classified subtypes (**Table 1**) and comprises the characteristics of "*proximal-distal non-antagonistic Co-C*". The explanation for the occurrence of this late Co-C lies most probably within the innervation pattern of the aforementioned muscles (**Figure 5**).

*Conclusion:* The recovered function of the greater pectoral muscle serves as an indicator of the likelihood of recovery of other distal muscles (forearm) of the upper extremity, which plays a leading role in co-activation pair; in this particular case, the greater pectoral muscle helped to navigate the contraction of ECRB and ECRL, providing not only clinically visible feedback, but also an EMG-assisted video-feedback during active rehabilitation. The increased power to ECRL/ECRB was only possible due to the helping assistance of the much earlier regenerated greater pectoral muscle.

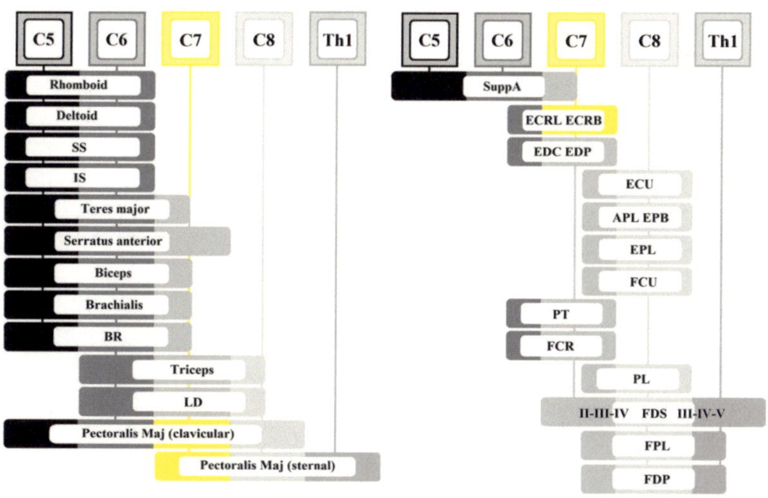


**Figure 5.**
*Schematic explanation of the occurrence of late proximal-distal Co-C (Pct-WE) associated with aberrant spontaneous regeneration of initially complete a-BPI (a similar color represents the same innervation pattern or root representation within the muscles and is most likely responsible for the emergence of co-contraction). SS—suprascapular muscle; IS—infrascapular muscle; BR—brachioradialis; LD—latissimus dorsi muscle; SuppA—supinator antebrachii muscle; ECRL—extensor carpi radialis longus; ECRB—Extensor carpi radialis brevis; EDC—Extensor digitorum communis; EDP—Extensor indicis and digiti minimi; ECU—Extensor carpi ulnaris; APL—Abductor pollicis brevis; EPB—Extensor pollicis brevis; EPL—extensor pollicis longus; FCU—flexor carpi ulnaris; PT—pronator teres muscle; FDS—flexor digitorum superficilalis; FPL—flexor pollicis longus; FDP—flexor digitorum profundus.*

### 3.3 Clinical example 3

A 33-year-old man was admitted to our department 5 mos. after a traction-type injury to the left brachial plexus in a motorcycle accident; neurological examination revealed non-functioning supraspinatus and infraspinatus, teres major and minor, deltoid and serratus anterior, biceps brachii (BB), coracobrachialis and brachialis muscles (0 points on the MRC scale—M0); latissimus dorsi muscle—M3; greater pectoral (Pct), all heads of triceps brachii (TB) muscles—M4; wrist (WE) and finger (FE) extensors—M4; wrist and finger flexors, intrinsics of the hand—M5. Clinically visible *aberrant spontaneous proximal-proximal non-antagonistic Co-C (Pct-TB)* and *aberrant spontaneous proximal-distal Co-C (TB-WE + FE)* were present. The projection of the innervation pattern to the muscles responsible for the occurrence of Co-C is shown in **Figure 6**.

The patient was diagnosed with cranially expanded C5-6 BPI, C4-5-6 avulsion was confirmed during the explorative surgery. The pool of available intraplexal motor donor nerves is shown in **Figure 6**.

In order to reanimate active elbow flexion, NT of ulnar nerve fascicles (m.flexor carpi ulnaris) to the musculocutaneous nerve (branches to biceps brachii muscle) or Oberlin 1 transfer was performed. Two other NTs were performed to reanimate flexion, abduction, and external rotation of the shoulder: Somsak [22, 23] and Bahm [21] NT, respectively.

Physiotherapy was resumed 6 weeks later. 15 mos. after surgery, shoulder flexion (sagittal plane), shoulder abduction (frontal plane), and external rotation were within normal ROM values. BB recovered to M4 and elbow flexion was near 90°, was independent. Hand function was severely impaired by the *induced*

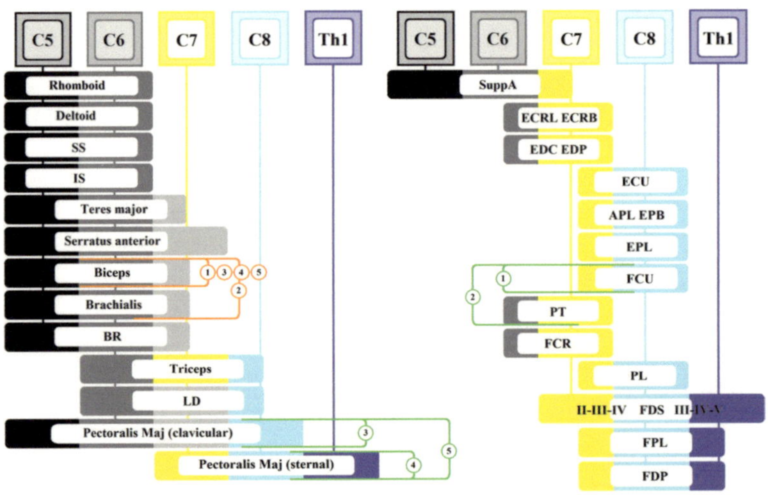


**Figure 6.**
*The pool of available intraplexal motor donor nerves in clinical example 3. Donor(s) are outlined in green; recipient(s) for the corresponding donornerves are outlined inorange: 1—ulnar nerve fascicles to m. flexor carpi ulnaris; 2—1 + proximal median nerve branch to m. pronator teres (double fascicular NT); 3 and 4—lateral and medial pectoral nerves respectively; 5—both lateral and medial pectoral nerves. *- injured roots are represented in black and gray; **—non-injured roots are represented in color; ***—similar color (thus, roots representation) represents same innervation-pattern of the muscles and is responsible, with great probability, for emergence of co-contraction; SS—suprascapular muscle; IS—infrascapular muscle; BR—brachioradialis; LD—latissimus dorsi muscle; SuppA—supinator antebrachii muscle; ECRL—extensor carpi radialis longus; ECRB—extensor carpi radialis brevis; EDC—extensor digitorum communis; EDP—extensor indicis and digiti minimi; ECU—extensor carpi ulnaris; APL—abductor pollicis brevis; EPB—extensor pollicis brevis; EPL—extensor pollicis longus; FCU—flexor carpi ulnaris; PT—pronator teres muscle; FDS—flexor digitorum superficilalis; FPL—flexor pollicis longus; FDP—flexor digitorum profundus.*

*proximal-distal Co-C (FCU/FDP4–5 + FCR-BB)* while pulling an object. *Aberrant spontaneous sequential proximal-distal Co-C (TB-WE + FE)* caused extension of the wrist and fingers while reaching the object (**Figure 7**). Wrist stability and the "opening/closing" of the hand were completely lost, the hand became non-functional.

*Pathology of biomechanics* (**Figure 8**): a "proximal co-contraction pool"—A (Pct and TB) becomes a kind of a 'trigger' for a "distal co-contraction pool"—C (FE and WE), which means that only sequential (in relation to elbow extension maneuver) wrist extension and hand opening is possible—a new "proximal-distal co-contraction pool"—B is formed. The "proximal co-contraction pool" dominates the "distal co-contraction pool" in a direct manner (proximal muscles act first). This type of

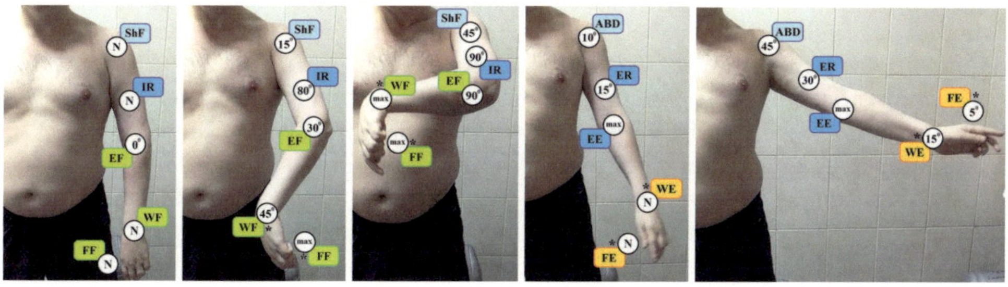


**Figure 7.**
*Correlation between BB function and wrist/finger biomechanics (proximal-distal* Co-C during active elbow flexion). ShF—shoulder flexion; ABD—shoulder abduction; IR—shoulder internal rotation; ER—external rotation; EF—elbow flexion; WE—wrist extension; FE—finger extension; N—neutral position; * Induced or regeneration associated proximal-distal Co-C.*

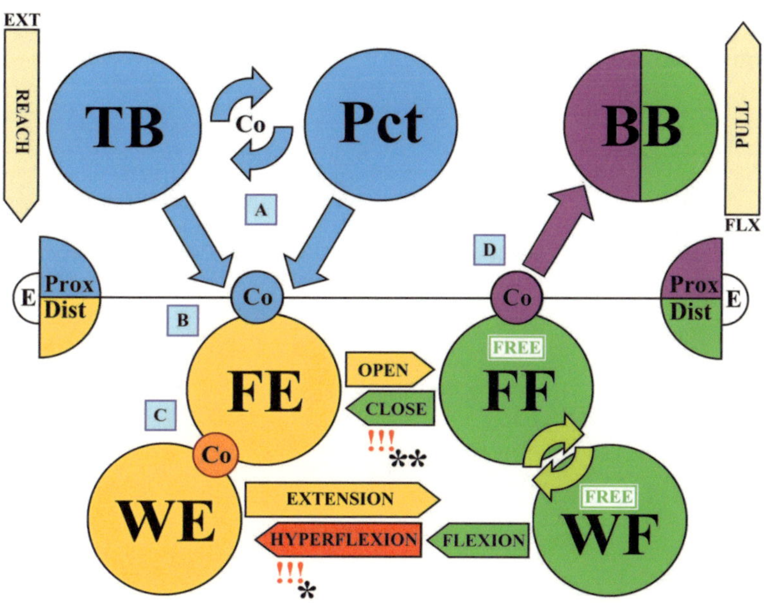


**Figure 8.**
*Function of proximal and distal segments of the upper extremity in case of BPI with Co-C following Oberlin or double-fascicular NT (hypothesis). EXT—elbow extension, reaching an object; FLX—elbow flexion, pulling an object; TB—triceps brachii muscle; Pct—greater pectoral muscle; BB—biceps brachii muscle; FE—finger extensors; WE—wrist extensors; FF—finger flexors; WF—wrist flexors; A—aberrant spontaneous non-antagonistic proximal-proximal Co-C; B—aberrant spontaneous proximal-distal sequential Co-C (arrow indicates the direction of action of primary Co-C initiator); C—aberrant spontaneous distal-distal sequential Co-C; D—induced proximal-distal Co-C (arrow indicates the direction of action of primary Co-C initiator); E—elbow; blue—primary co-contractors; green—independent movement; both colors—partially independent. *—Aggravation of wrist flexion; **—aggravation of finger flexion.*

co-activation does not disturb the global function in relation to the direction of the entire action of the upper limb reaching an object. Surgical reconstruction of active elbow flexion through Oberlin 1 nerve transfer leads to the emergence of a new form of a "proximal-distal co-contraction pool"—D (FF and BB). Hence, the activation of BB depends on activation of FF (serve as a 'trigger'), the newly emerged co-contraction pool becomes more of a distal-proximal type, where FFs dominate in reverse order (distal muscles act first). This type of co-activation does not disturb the global function in relation to the direction of the entire action of the upper limb pulling an object. As a result, the proximal muscles (above the elbow joint), primary antagonists, BB, and TB can act independently. At the same time, the distal muscles (below the elbow joint), primary antagonists, WE/WF and FE/FF are unable to act independently during basic activities of daily living (ADLs). For instance, reaching the face, mouth, contralateral axillary groove while holding an object (cup, toothbrush, deodorant) requires elbow flexion and at least wrist stability or slight extension. Knowing that the initiator of wrist extension (WE) acts in the opposite direction (TB), their primary function to stabilize the wrist joint is lost, which leads to hyperfunction of FF and WF as initiators of elbow flexion, and finally, to the wrist and finger hyperflexion.

*Short rational explanation:* Pulling an object when the elbow flexion is done activates the cortical centers of the finger and wrist flexors (Oberlin effect or phenomenon) which leads to wrist and finger hyperflexion. The inability to use the wrist extensors as a compensatory mechanism is related to their activation only when the extremity moves in the opposite direction, the elbow extends when reaching an object.

*Conclusion: Induced* and *spontaneous proximal-distal and distal-proximal Co-C* are confronting each other, this confrontation disables hand opening/closing during principal basic ADLs. We do not recommend utilizing the Oberlin 1 transfer in similar cases.

This clinical example reflects the *pro* and *contra* arguments of using available fascicles of the ulnar nerve as a donor in case of a-BPI accompanied by aberrant spontaneous proximal-distal Co-C (**Table 2**).

| PRO | CONTRA |
|---|---|
| Oberlin NT could potentially lead to BB recovery with power exceeding M4 and, without confronting function of TB, could possibly produce higher degree of elbow flexion. | Basically, patients without aberrant spontaneous Co-C compensate for the inability to dissociate movements in the proximal and distal segments (the Oberlin phenomenon or effect [8] in almost one-third of cases [6]) with an independent function of wrist extensors, which provides stability and helps to avoid hyperflexion in the wrist joint when reaching (elbow extension) and pulling (elbow flexion) an object. The main contra argument against Oberlin is the occurrence of *induced proximal-distal Co-C (BB and WF/FF)* that severely aggravates on the basis of complete loss of independent wrist extension due to *aberrant spontaneous proximal-distal Co-C (TB and WE/FE).* |

**Table 2.**
*Pro and contra arguments of utilizing the ulnar nerve fascicles in case of a-BPI accompanied by aberrant spontaneous proximal-distal Co-C.*

### 3.4 Clinical example 4

A 37-year-old man was admitted to our department 7 mos. after traction-type injury to left brachial plexus in a motorcycle accident; neurological examination revealed non-functioning supraspinatus and infraspinatus muscles, teres major and minor, deltoid and serratus anterior, biceps brachii (BB), coracobrachialis and brachialis muscles (0 points on the MRC scale—M0); latissimus dorsi muscle—M3; greater pectoral (Pct), all heads of triceps brachii (TB) muscles—M4; wrist (WE) and finger (FE) extensors—M4; wrist and finger flexors, intrinsics of the hand—M5. Clinically visible *aberrant spontaneous proximal-proximal non-antagonistic Co-C (Pct-TB)* and *aberrant spontaneous*

*DOI: http://dx.doi.org/10.5772/intechopen.100609*

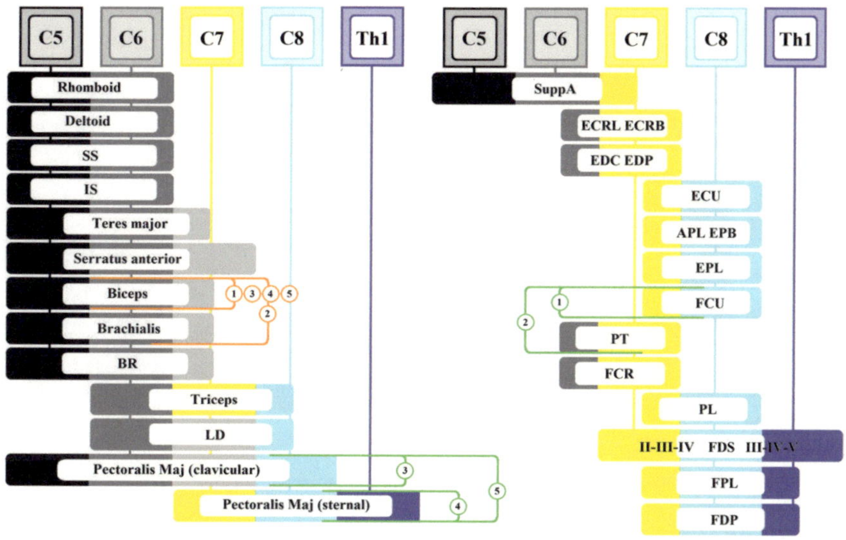


**Figure 9.**
*Pool of available intraplexal motor donor nerves in clinical example 4. Donor(s) are outlined in green; recipient(s) for the corresponding donor nerves are outlined in orange): 1—ulnar nerve fascicles to m. flexor carpi ulnaris; 2—1 + proximal median nerve branch to m. pronator teres (double fascicular NT); 3 and 4—lateral and medial pectoral nerves, respectively; 5—both lateral and medial pectoral nerves. *—Injured roots are shown in black and gray; **—intact roots are represented in color; ***—a similar color (thus, the representation of roots) represents same innervationpattern of muscles and is most likely responsible for theemergence of co-contraction; SS—suprascapular muscle; IS—infrascapular muscle; BR—brachioradialis; LD—latissimus dorsi muscle; SuppA—supinator antebrachii muscle; ECRL—extensor carpi radialis longus; ECRB—extensor carpi radialis brevis; EDC—extensor digitorum communis; EDP—extensor indicis and digiti minimi; ECU—extensor carpi ulnaris; APL—abductor pollicis brevis; EPB—extensor pollicis brevis; EPL—extensor pollicis longus; FCU—flexor carpi ulnaris; PT—pronator teres muscle; FDS—flexor digitorum superficialis; FPL—flexor pollicis longus; FDP—flexor digitorum profundus.*

*proximal-distal Co-C (TB-WE + FE)* were present. The projection of the innervation pattern of the muscles responsible for the occurrence of Co-C is shown in **Figure 9**.

The patient was diagnosed with cranially expanded C5-6 BPI, C4-5-6 avulsion was confirmed during the explorative surgery. The pool of available intraplexal motor donor nerves is shown in **Figure 9**.

In order to reanimate active elbow flexion, there was performed an NT of medial pectoral to musculocutaneous nerve distally to the branches of the coracobrachialis muscle. Two other NTs were performed to reanimate flexion, abduction, and external rotation of the shoulder: Somsak [22, 23] and Bahm [21] NT, respectively.

Physiotherapy was resumed 6 weeks later. 14 mos. after the surgery, abduction of the shoulder in the frontal plane was 75°, external rotation was 20°. BB recovered to M3 and elbow flexion was near 40°. Elbow flexion was severely burdened by the conversion from *aberrant spontaneous proximal-proximal non-antagonistic Co-C (Pct-TB)* to *induced proximal-proximal antagonistic Co-C (BB-TB)*. The clinical picture was dominated by "triceps syndrome".

The injection of botulinum toxin A at the appropriate dose into the long head of the TB was performed. Significant weakening of the long head of the TB was observed 3 mos. after injection. Physiotherapy proceeded and 19 mos. after surgery, the power of BB increased to M4, elbow flexion increased to 90° and BB became partially independent (**Figure 10**). *Aberrant spontaneous proximal-distal Co-C (TB-WE + FE)* remained disturbing and complicated the utilization of the non-dominant upper extremity during daily occupations.

*Pathology of biomechanics* (**Figure 11**): the pre-surgical "proximal co-contraction pool"—A (Pct and TB) becomes a kind of "trigger" for the "distal co-contraction

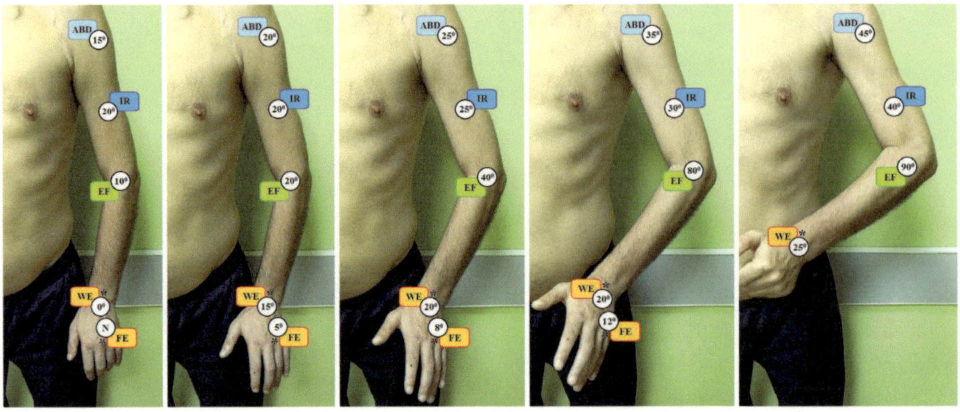


**Figure 10.**
*Correlation between BB function and wrist/finger biomechanics (proximal-distal* Co-C during active elbow flexion). ABD—shoulder abduction; IR—shoulder internal rotation; EF—elbow flexion; WE—wrist extension; FE—finger extension; N—neutral position.*

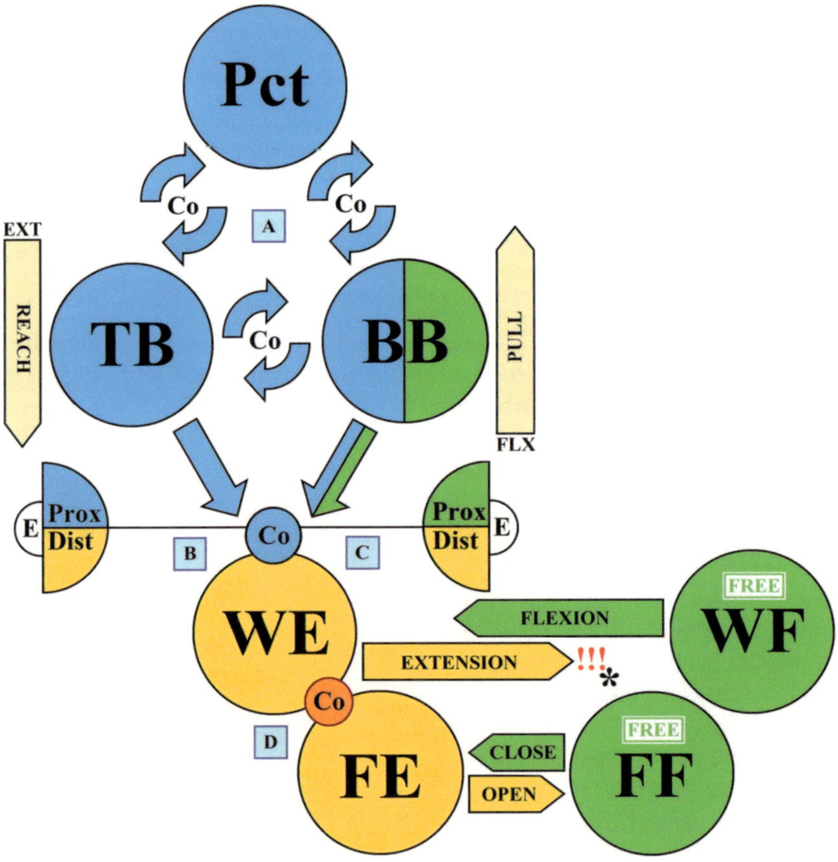


**Figure 11.**
*Function of proximal and distal segments of the upper extremity in case of BPI with Co-C following medial pectoral to musculocutaneous NT (result). TB—triceps brachii muscle; Pct—greater pectoral muscle; BB—biceps brachii muscle; FE—finger extensors; WE—wrist extensors; FF—finger flexors; WF—wrist flexors; A—aberrant spontaneous non-antagonistic proximal-proximal and induced antagonistic proximal-proximal Co-C; B—aberrant spontaneous proximal-distal sequential Co-C (arrow indicates the direction of action of primary Co-C initiator); C—aberrant spontaneous proximal-distal sequential Co-C associated with elbow flexion (arrow indicates the direction of action of primary Co-C initiator); D—aberrant spontaneous distal-distal sequential Co-C; E—elbow; blue—primary co-contractors; green—independent movement; both colors—partially independent. *—Aggravation of wrist extension.*

pool"—D (FE and WE), which means that only sequential (in relation to the elbow extension maneuver) wrist extension and opening of the hand is possible, a new "proximal-distal co-contraction pool"—B is formed. The "proximal co-contraction pool" dominates the "distal co-contraction pool" in a direct manner (proximal muscles act first). This type of co-activation does not disturb the global function in relation to the direction of the entire upper limb action reaching an object. Surgical reconstruction of active elbow flexion through medial pectoral NT results in the introduction of a new member in the "proximal co-contraction pool" BB. The post-surgical/post-recovery "proximal co-contraction pool"—A—now consists of Pct, TB and BB. As a result, the proximal muscles (above the elbow joint), the primary antagonists, BB and TB could not act independently. Temporary "switching-off" of TB, the primary BB antagonist, leads to partial independence of BB. The "proximal co-contraction pool" still dominates the "distal co-contraction pool" in a direct manner (proximal muscles act first). This type of co-activation does not disturb the global function in relation to the direction of the entire upper limb action both when pulling and reaching an object. The distal muscles (below the elbow joint), the primary antagonist, WE/WF and FE/FF are able to act independently during the basic activities of daily living (ADLs), allowing the hand to open or to close freely. For instance, reaching the face, mouth, and contralateral axillary groove while holding an object (cup, toothbrush, and deodorant) requires elbow flexion and at least wrist stability or minor extension. Knowing that the TB, the initiator of wrist extension (WE), acts simultaneously with BB (both from the same new "co-contraction pool") their primary function of stabilizing the wrist joint is preserved whether during reaching (elbow extension) or pulling (elbow flexion) an object.

*Short rational explanation:* Pulling an object with the elbow flexion simultaneously activates the cortical centers of the triceps brachii muscle, as well as the wrist and finger extensors. Partial independence of the biceps brachii muscle is most probably related to the "drifting" of the cortical center of the elbow flexion. The inability to completely dissociate the muscles of the "proximal co-contraction pool" (TB, BB, B) is reflected in the power and angular performance rate of the biceps brachii muscle. The co-existence of confronting *proximal Co-C* upon reaching and pulling an object with elbow flexion/extension has only a minor influence on wrist flexion/extension, hand opening/closing, while the preexisting *proximal-distal Co-C* enables physiologic wrist positioning during ADLs.

*Conclusion:* Regardless of the fact that we obtained only 90° of the elbow flexion with medial pectoral NT and the confronting function of TB partially disabled independent elbow flexion, the distal segments of the upper extremity remained highly functional.

This clinical example reflects the *pro* and *contra* arguments of the utilization of an available medial pectoral donor nerve in case of BPI accompanied by aberrant spontaneous proximal-distal Co-C (**Table 3**).

| PRO | CONTRA |
|---|---|
| The conversion of *aberrant spontaneous non-antagonistic proximal-proximal Co-C (Pct-TB) into induced antagonistic proximal-proximal Co-C (BB-TB)* did not produce confronting Co-Cs during reaching and pulling an object only in the distal segments of the upper extremity. As a result, the main pro argument in favor of the provided NT is that it does not disturb the independent hand opening. Wrist hyperextension that accompanies either reaching or pulling an object is compensated for the independent function of the wrist flexors. | The conversion of the *aberrant spontaneous non-antagonistic proximal-proximal Co-C (Pct-TB) into induced antagonistic proximal-proximal Co-C (BB-TB)* produces confronting Co-Cs during reaching and pulling an object in the proximal segment of the upper extremity. As a result, BB becomes partially independent of TB, yet the confronting. Co-C between TB and BB prevents BB from executing its full flexion potential in the elbow joint. Regardless the fact that BB power reaches M4, the elbow flexion does not exceed 90° |

**Table 3.**
*Pro and contra arguments of utilization of the medial pectoral nerve in case of a-BPI accompanied by aberrant spontaneous proximal-distal Co-C.*

## 4. Summary

We believe that, regardless of all existing limitations, we provide an interesting insight in terms of a compromise solution for a specific case of BPI accompanied by Co-Cs of different types. The study of the natural history of the individual regeneration process, a thorough preoperative evaluation of *pros* and *contras,* and advantages and disadvantages of available NTs, lead to the emergence of a reconstruction plan that allows not only to expand the functions of the upper arm (restore elbow flexion), but also not to disturb the pre-existing partially pathological, yet highly functional, biomechanics of wrist and fingers, to improve the overall function of the entire upper extremity.

## Author details

Alexander A. Gatskiy* and Ihor B. Tretyak
The State Institution "Romodanov Neurosurgery Institute of National Academy of Medical Sciences of Ukraine", Kyiv, Ukraine

*Address all correspondence to: drgatskiy@outlook.com

## References

[1] Kline DG. Timing for brachial plexus injury: A personal experience. Neurosurgery Clinics of North America. 2009;**20**(1):24-26

[2] Giuffre JL, Kakar S, Bishop AT, Spinner RJ, Shin AY. Current concepts of the treatment of adult brachial plexus injuries. Journal of Hand Surgery. 2010;**35**(4):678-688

[3] Martin E, Senders JT, DiRisio AC, Smith TR, Broekman MLD. Timing of surgery in traumatic brachial plexus injury: A systematic review. Journal of Neurosurgery. 2018;**1**:1-13

[4] Socolovsky M, Costales JR, Paez MD, Nizzo G, Valbuena S, Varone E. Obstetric brachial plexus palsy: Reviewing the literature comparing the results of primary versus secondary surgery. Child's Nervous System. 2015;**32**(3):415-425

[5] Noetzel MJ, Wolpaw JR. Emerging concepts in the pathophysiology of recovery from neonatal brachial plexus injury. Neurology. 2000;**55**(1):5-6

[6] Brown T, Cupido C, Scarfone H, Pape K, Galea V, McComas A. Developmental apraxia arising from neonatal brachial plexus palsy. Neurology. 2000;**55**(1):24-30

[7] Arad E, Stephens D, Curtis CG, Clarke HM. Botulinum toxin for the treatment of motor imbalance in obstetrical brachial plexus palsy. Plastic and Reconstructive Surgery. 2013; **131**(6):1307-1315

[8] Hems T. Nerve transfers for traumatic brachial plexus injury: Advantages and problems. Journal of Hand and Microsurgery. 2016;**03**(1):6-10

[9] Hesselmans LF, Jennekens FG, Van den Oord CJ, Veldman H, Vincent A. Development of innervation of skeletal muscle fibers in man: Relation to acetylcholine receptors. The Anatomical Record. 1993;**236**(3):553-562

[10] Gramsbergen A, van Eykern LA, Meek MF. Sciatic nerve transection in adult and young rats: Abnormal EMG patterns during locomotion. Equine Veterinary Journal Supplement. 2001;**33**:36-40

[11] Esslen E. Electromyographic findings on two types of misdirection of regenerating axons. Electroencephalography and Clinical Neurophysiology. 1960;**12**(738-741):1960

[12] Brandt KE, Mackinnon SE. A technique for maximizing biceps recovery in brachial plexus reconstruction. Journal of Hand Surgery. 1993;**18**(4):726-733

[13] Shin YB, Shin MJ, Chang JH, Cha YS, Ko HY. Effects of botulinum toxin on reducing the co-contraction of antagonists in birth brachial plexus palsy. Annals of Rehabilitation Medicine. 2014;**38**(1):127

[14] Chuang DC. Debates to personal conclusion in peripheral nerve injury and reconstruction: A 30-year experience at Chang Gung Memorial Hospital. Indian Journal of Plastic Surgery. 2016;**49**(2):144

[15] Oberlin C, Béal D, Leechavengvongs S, Salon A, Dauge MC, Sarcy JJ. Nerve transfer to biceps muscle using a part of ulnar nerve for C5–C6 avulsion of the brachial plexus: Anatomical study and report of four cases. Journal of Hand Surgery. 1994;**19**(2):232-237

[16] Mackinnon SE, Novak CB, Myckatyn TM, Tung TH. Results of reinnervation of the biceps and brachialis muscles with a double fascicular transfer for elbow flexion.

Journal of Hand Surgery. 2005;**30**(5): 978-985

[17] Escudero RB, Rezende MR, Wataya EY, Pontes FV, Cho ÁB, Pisani MJ. Correlation between the elbow flexion and the hand and wrist flexion after neurotization of the fascicles of the ulnar nerve to the motor branch to the biceps. Revista Brasileira de Ortopedia. 2017;**52**(3):309-314

[18] Ray WZ, Mackinnon SE. Clinical outcomes following median to radial nerve transfers. Journal of Hand Surgery. 2011;**36**(2):201-208

[19] Siqueira MG, Martins RS. Surgical treatment of adult traumatic brachial plexus injuries. Arquivos de Neuro-Psiquiatria. 2011;**69**(3):528-535

[20] Dvali L, Mackinnon S. Nerve repair, grafting, and nerve transfers. Clinics in Plastic Surgery. 2003;**30**(2):203-221

[21] Bahm J, Noaman H, Becker M. The dorsal approach to the suprascapular nerve in neuromuscular reanimation for obstetric brachial plexus lesions. Plastic and Reconstructive Surgery. 2005; **115**(1):240-244

[22] Witoonchart K, Leechavengvongs S, Uerpairojkit C, Thuvasethakul P, Wongnopsuwan V. Nerve transfer to deltoid muscle using the nerve to the long head of the triceps, part I: An anatomic feasibility study. The Journal of Hand Surgery. 2003;**28**(4):628-632

[23] Leechavengvongs S, Witoonchart K, Uerpairojkit C, Thuvasethakul P. Nerve transfer to deltoid muscle using the nerve to the long head of the triceps, part II: A report of 7 cases. The Journal of Hand Surgery. 2003;**28**(4):633-638

Chapter 10

# Frontiers of Brachial Plexus Injury: Future Revolutions in the Field

*Joseph M. Rosen, Jennifer Hong, Julien Klaudt-Moreau, Allison Podsednik and Vincent R. Hentz*

## Abstract

The field of brachial plexus surgery has undergone dramatic changes in the past 40 years. Most of these have been incremental in nature. We have seen increased use of nerve grafts and nerve transfers. We have seen the introduction of robotic limb replacements for the most severe flail limbs where surgical intervention has failed. In some cases, we have seen an increase in the use of computer simulation and virtual reality to train surgeons to plan and execute surgeries. More recently, we have seen the introduction of technologies derived from regenerative medicine research.

However, we expect to see a true revolution in the field of brachial plexus surgery in the next 40 years, specifically:

- We anticipate an increasing introduction of biotechnologies from regenerative medicine.

- We expect fundamental changes in our understanding of nerve repair and the introduction of Fusogens allowing us to couple nerve ends, establishing immediate functional connections, and avoiding distal Wallerian degeneration.

- We will be able to prevent atrophy of muscles distal to nerve injury and accelerate axonal regeneration.

- We will also see a comprehensive understanding in the mechanism of apoptosis of the distal peripheral segment, and brain and spinal cord neurons proximal to the injury, leading to pharmacological manipulation of the mitochondria and other organelles in the distal nerve from signaling cell death and therefore interrupting the normal cascade that leads to Wallerian degeneration.

- In chronic brachial plexus injuries where the limb musculature has irreversibly atrophied, we will have three choices – robotic replacements, limb transplantation and limb regeneration. However, the most likely solution will be robotics in the near future.

- We will see a revolution in both the design and control of robotic limbs through brain-machine interfaces. Computers will allow us through virtual reality to model the brachial plexus in extreme detail. These simulation models will enable the prediction of outcomes of our surgery. Detailed physically-based models of the injury obtained pre-operatively will allow us to better plan for surgery. Bringing these models into the operating room (through augmented reality) creates a "performance machine" enabling us to better see and manipulate the brachial plexus as we operate by superimposing our living models on the patient's anatomy.

- In the more distant future, we will repair nerves by actually guiding axon connections, recreating normal neuro-muscular and neuro-sensory architecture.

All of these advances will revolutionize the practice of brachial plexus surgery and ultimately result in truly improved outcomes for our patients with the most devastating brachial plexus injuries.

> *"The dreams of yesterday are the hopes of today and the reality of tomorrow."*[1] — *Robert H. Goddard — father of the US space program*
>
> *At the time of this quote, Robert Goddard was sitting in a tree in his backyard as a high school student — and a true visionary. He believed we would reach the moon and beyond, and he later created the original ideas that the space program was founded on for the next century.*

**Keywords:** brachial plexus surgery, nerve grafts, robotic limbs, simulation, virtual reality, tissue engineering, regenerative medicine

## 1. Introduction

### 1.1 The last 40 years – Seeing further by standing on the shoulders of giants

Over the last 40 years, the field of brachial plexus surgery has greatly advanced. We have moved from a field with initial poor outcomes to one that is now able to provide hope to our patients. In many cases, our successes have changed a useless limb into a functional assistive limb. In occasional cases, we have restored almost-normal function to paralyzed limbs. However, in the most severe injuries, such as those resulting in a chronic flail arm, we continue to struggle with failure to improve outcomes. We have seen a wide adoption of new surgical techniques, first introduced in the latter half of the 20th century, which are now common practice in the daily treatment of patients with brachial plexus injuries. These techniques have been applied to patients in all stages of life, from birth defects to adult brachial plexus injuries. They include microsurgery, autologous and artificial nerve grafting, and tissue engineering to fabricate nerve conduits. Sophisticated surgical techniques including vascularized nerve grafts and functional muscle transfers have been developed and successfully applied. We have seen the use of nerve transfers, initially performed in selected cases, become the standard of care for some conditions, and in many clinical scenarios we have switched from an operative approach of repair of a very proximal injury to creating distal nerve transfers that more rapidly restore functional outcomes. Indeed, the rising popularity of nerve transfers has led to testing and validation of a variety of donor sites – including contralateral nerve roots and intercostals – with new ones being introduced and tested almost every year.

In the most severe chronic injuries when conventional surgery has failed, patients often accept amputation. In these cases, the distal limb muscles have atrophied and vthe limb has become a burdensome "parasite." For patients with a chronically denervated extremity, a robotic limb that can be controlled through myoelectric

[1] https://quotefancy.com/quote/1669979/Robert-H-Goddard-The-dreams-of-yesterday-are-the-hopes-of-today-and-the-reality-of

interfaces can be a dramatic improvement. Robotic technology has experienced a revolution in its capabilities to produce durable artificial hands with fully functional five-finger dexterity, and the materials and methodologies for their manufacture. We have seen the increasing clinical use of brain-machine interfaces to address neurological problems resulting in advances that can now be translated into use for artificial limbs. Many patients have received transplanted limbs; a technology that eventually could be applied to the most severe chronic brachial plexus injured limbs. The safety of whole-limb allotransplantation has improved with new immunosuppression protocols; however, donor limb supply still remains a major limitation. Although regenerative medicine has provided many solutions in multiple fields, the complete regeneration of a limb remains beyond the scope of this chapter. Even with the increased interest in total-limb regeneration in invertebrates and a few amphibians and the introduction of new tools of genetic engineering like CRISPR, it is unlikely that we will be able to manipulate our own genome to restore a limb in our Lifetime.

The realistic advances expected over the next 40 years will be driven largely by today's unanswered needs and questions. What is lacking today are the answers to clinical gaps that include:

- Lack of technologies that accurately assess the injured nerve roots and provide a detailed prognosis for recovery – we need sophisticated preoperative electrodiagnostic tools that map the injury and intraoperative imaging to guide the surgeon.
- Lack of nerve grafts – we need substitutes that are even better than autografts, that contain the right structural matrix and cells with already "up-regulated" genes.
- Slow pace of axonal growth – we need methods to speed axonal growth, or somehow obviate the need for axonal regeneration after nerve transection and repair or reconstruction.
- Nerve degeneration distal to the injury – we need protective molecules or technologies that either slow the pace of – or better, prevent – Wallerian degeneration of the axons distal to the site of injury.
- Inability to accurately connect proximal and distal axons at the site of nerve repair – we need to not only re-establish the nerve connections between the proximal and distal ends but also correctly connect proximal individual axons to the exactly corresponding distal axons. That would require nerve repair not at the epineural level, or at the fascicle level, but at the axon level – the true level that is needed for successful functional recovery [1].

## 2. Part I: Acute injuries and their treatment, now and in the future

### 2.1 Regenerative medicine: Augmenting the healing process

There has been a revolution in regenerative medicine in the past two decades (**Figure 1**). We have seen the ability to control human stem cells and transform them into almost every type of adult cell including the peripheral nervous system [2]. Today, regenerative medicine and tissue engineering allow us to grow human nerve grafts. Tissue-engineered nerve grafts (TENGs) have been developed and transplanted into large animal models to span large gaps [3, 4]. As allograft development has progressed, the scaffolds and materials available for nerve repair have provided functional outcomes for patients that are comparable to the existing gold-standard autograft [5]. Allografts also have the potential to exceed the ability of autografts to facilitate nerve regeneration, as they are capable of being modified

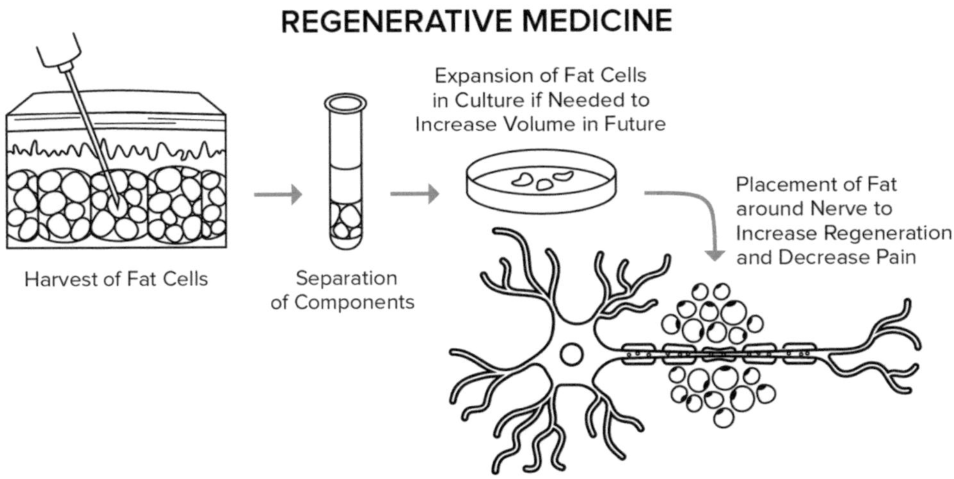


**Figure 1.**
*Regenerative Medicine (Section 2.1). Cells (such as fat cells) are harvested and processed to concentrate the stem cells or grow them in culture. The cells are then injected around the nerve injury site, a process that has several roles: to assist in nerve regeneration and to decrease neuropathic pain. The cells act at the injury site and also at the proximal axon and cell body and further proximally in the spinal cord.*

with pro-regenerative growth factors, impregnated with patient-derived stem-cells, and be structurally engineered to prevent axon misdirection [6–10].

We have seen the beginnings of a shift from autografts to allografts and can anticipate the common adoption of totally artificial, tissue-engineered substitutes. These will be a combination of scaffolds, key bioagents, and cell components. Widespread use of allografts that can improve on the functional outcomes of autografts is highly desirable as these biomaterials will reduce patient pain and disability from surgery to harvest autografts, increase the amount of graft material available to reconstruct long gaps in large nerves, and decrease operative time overall. Due to regulatory pathways of the Food and Drug Administration (FDA) and other agencies, there are many hurdles to overcome in the introduction of these stem-cell types, [11] whether derived from fetal cells or from the transformation of adult cells.

A second area of active interest in regenerative medicine is the use of stem cells to promote growth and speed healing. Mesenchymal stem cells are pluripotent cells that persist into adulthood, and can be found in bone marrow and adipose tissue. These cells can support nerve regeneration through multiple functions including secretion of growth factors such as vascular endothelial growth factor (VEGF), differentiate into progenitor cells, and modulate the inflammatory response [12–15]. At present, there is a growing use of adipose stem cells which are more abundant than bone-marrow stem cells and easily harvested in the operating room for peripheral nerve surgery [16] and several other orthopedic applications, including injection into joints and around tendons to encourage function and decrease pain. Fat cells are used to prevent scarred nerves that have been surgically freed from re-forming scars. Fat cells are also used to prevent neuropathic pain and encourage nerve regeneration [17]. They have been increasingly used in the past 10 years and we expect their use to expand in the next 40 years.

We can also expect to see regenerative medicine create nerve–muscle units. Much of this work is already being done successfully in many laboratories for small muscles such as the intrinsic muscles in the hand. In some cases, muscle is being grown to replace muscle that has been lost in limbs from blast injuries in wounded warriors. We expect these new biomaterials to become part of our armamentarium in brachial plexus injuries where distal muscle loss could be replaced with key nerve-muscle regenerated substitutes [18].

### *2.1.1 Tissue-engineered nerve grafts (TENGs) (additional reading)*

These additional readings include an overview of peripheral nerve repair approaches used [19] and further delve into TENGs including their efficacy, [20] advances, [21] and interactions with native tissue [22].

| Reference | Topic overview |
|---|---|
| [19] | A review of peripheral nerve repair approaches including hydrogel fillers, fibrous interluminal fillers, and interluminal scaffolds |
| [20] | A study investigating the efficacy of living vs. nonliving scaffolds in peripheral nerve repair |
| [21] | A review of the advances and efficacy of TENGs including recent modifications and enhancements to the scaffolds |
| [22] | A review paper examining the two-way interactions between native cellular tissues and electrospun matricies that serve as tissue scaffolds |

## 2.2 Fusogens: Shifting the paradigm of nerve repair

Fusogens are a key innovation in peripheral nerve surgery. Fusogens are chemicals that allow cell membranes, which normally repel each other, to fuse together. In the context of nerve injury, they allow for fusion of the cell membranes enclosing the two severed ends of the axon, thus establishing continuity at the cellular level between the proximal and distal nerve. They are a paradigm shift in our thinking and approach to nerve injuries. Our surgical approaches have previously focused on fixing nerve discontinuity by suturing the epineurium of severed nerves together. This intervention fails to act on the underlying cellular structures that are affected by injury, namely the axon. By overcoming the inherent molecular barriers to axon continuity, fusogens offer a new therapeutic avenue for treating and rapidly healing acute nerve transections. This technology was not considered possible prior to the new millennium, but in the past two decades there has been an increasing accumulation of evidence that not only can invertebrates fuse proximal and distal divided axons, but we can also create the condition in vertebrates [23] to allow fusion to occur in both spinal cord [24] and peripheral nerve injuries [25]. Since 2000, there has been an explosion of different fusogen chemicals that would allow severed proximal axonal membranes to re-connect to distal axonal membranes [26] in the timeframe before Wallerian degeneration occurs [27]. Within the first 72 hours after a nerve transection, the axon membrane of the proximal axon and the axon membrane of the distal stump could be successfully fused in vertebrates (**Figure 2**). It was not clear what the mechanism for this fusion was, or what was the best pharmacological agent to encourage fusion. With this initial success in the peripheral nervous system of vertebrates, interest grew to move forward and at the present time fusogens are being used in clinical trials for digital nerve injuries [28, 29].

Fusogens are currently under investigation for clinical use in humans, using a digital nerve repair model. They have not yet been used for brachial plexus injuries, but their application to the brachial plexus would be very significant. The major limitation of brachial plexus injuries is the long distance from the injury site to the distal end organs, especially the motor units. By the time the regenerating axons reach the target muscles, significant muscle atrophy has transpired. A reconstructive alternative to nerve repair, nerve transfers, when possible, can significantly shorten regenerative times and re-establish myoneural junctions. This approach,

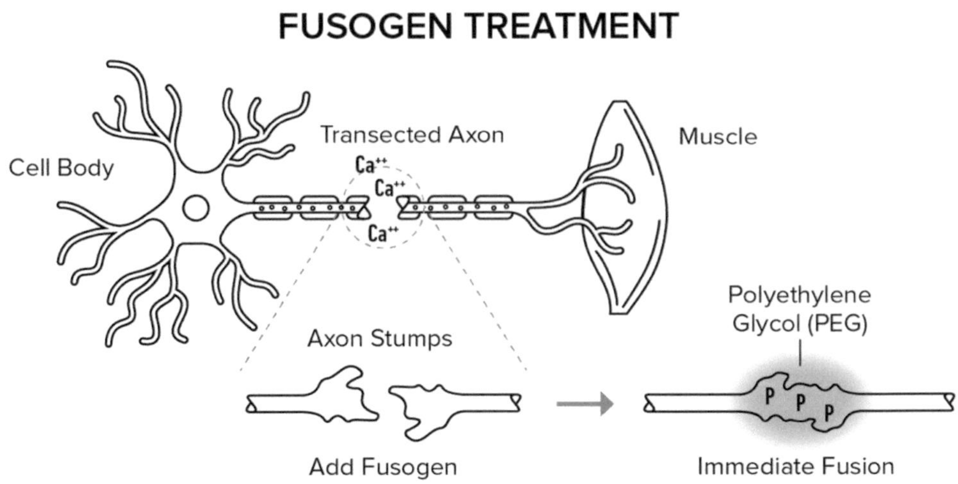


**Figure 2.**
*Fusogen Treatment (Section 2.2). Fusogens act at the repair site to enable the cytoplasm of the proximal and distal axon to immediately fuse after being transected. The most commonly used fusogen at the present time is polyethylene glycol (PEG). The mechanism of action is not presently known but PEG is thought to act directly on the cytoplasmic membranes at the time of injury to enable them to fuse. PEG stabilizes the physical chemistry and properties of the membranes, enabling them to fuse through the biological-chemical interactions with the multiple layers of the cytoplasmic membranes and the influence of their surfactant properties.*

when used in concert with a fusogen, could potentially provide immediate re-establishment of axon continuity and electrical conductivity. This would prevent the atrophy [30] seen in brachial plexus injuries. We are now at the beginning of clinical trials for digital nerves. This is the first test of this vast change in peripheral nerve surgery. We would then expect to see applications to larger mixed nerves such as the median and ulnar nerve at the wrist and then more proximal nerves. Eventually it could be applied to the most proximal brachial plexus injuries where it is clearly most needed.

In the next section, we discuss how to keep the distal nerve alive so that it would be available for a fusogen solution or just a conventional nerve repair. This would greatly increase the number of cases in which a fusogen could be used to instantaneously restore axon continuity and function.

### *2.2.1 "State-of-the-art nerve transfers" (additional reading)*

In these additional readings, one can learn more information regarding nerve transfer including their uses, [31, 32] suggested adjunct procedures, [32] efficacy and outcomes, [33] and comparison to nerve grafts [34].

| Reference | Topic overview |
|---|---|
| [31] | A review investigating the use of distal nerve transfers to the ulnar nerve in cubital tunnel syndrome |
| [32] | A review of nerve transfer use in peripheral nerve injury and suggestion of concomitant Schwann cell transplantation to aid in regeneration |
| [33] | A systematic review assessing the efficacy and outcome correlations of nerve transfer in patients with brachial plexus and axillary nerve injury |
| [34] | A systematic review evaluating nerve graft vs. nerve transfer regarding shoulder abduction recovery in patients with brachial plexus palsy |

### 2.3 Apoptosis: The role of the mitochondria and other organelles in axonal death

Fusogens require a viable distal nerve to work. In most brachial plexus injuries, it is not possible to intervene before the distal nerve experiences Wallerian degeneration. Once the process of distal degeneration has begun, fusion of the membranes of the proximal and distal axons is no longer possible. However, in the past decade significant strides have been made in our understanding of the process of apoptosis – the cascade that initiates cell death and in the peripheral nerve, the process that initiates the loss of the distal axon. Through recent experimental work in vertebrate animal models, it is clear that organelles in the distal axon initiate apoptosis. In particular, the mitochondria play an overwhelming role in this process. Mitochondria were once a form or bacteria that invaded cells and then became a crucial part of the cell's metabolism responsible for energy production for the eukaryote cell. In the axon, there are several types of mitochondria – some that migrate and others that are relatively stationary [9, 35]. At the site of nerve injury, a calcium wave is propagated down the distal axon. The mitochondria are directly affected by this calcium wave. The mitochondria have an outside membrane wall and an inner membrane wall. The calcium wave causes a state of increased permeability of the outer membrane of the mitochondria [36]. The outer membrane of the mitochondria is contributed by the host cell and the inner mitochondrial membrane is a part of the original primordial mitochondria before it became a part of the cell or in this case the axon.

The state of increased permeability of the outer membrane is key to the initiation of the cascade that ultimately results in the signaling of cell death. The mitochondria release proteins in the form of enzymes that begins apoptosis. This then signals and engages the Schwann cells to transform into Bungner tubes. The Schwann cells then recruit monocytes, and the monocytes transform into macrophages that play a crucial role in engulfing the debris of the distal axon in the process of Wallerian degeneration.

What if we could interrupt the cascade of apoptosis initiated by the mitochondria? It has been shown through pharmacological means that molecules of certain dimensions [36] can block the permeability of the outer membrane caused by the calcium wave after nerve injury, whether by crush or transection. For example, molecules of polyethylene glycol (PEG) can be introduced and selectively block the pores in the outer membrane of the distal axon mitochondria and thus block apoptosis [27, 37]. This would provide a kind of immortality for the distal axon (**Figure 3**). If the distal axon remains viable, then this opens up key opportunities in the repair of nerves after a brachial plexus injury. Viable distal axons could be fused to proximal axons through the introduction of fusogens at the transection site, causing an immediate reconnection of the proximal and distal stumps and the immediate reestablishment of connectivity, and most importantly, conductivity of action potentials [38]. This would prevent the distal end organs from atrophying, [30] and allow the muscles to remain viable and functional through the connections with their distal axons across the myoneural junctions [39]. In addition, viable distal axons would allow nerve repair even without fusogens. The proximal nerve stump axons with their activated mitochondria will send out growth cones that will enter the distal axon and re-establish connectivity. There would be no distal Wallerian degeneration because the distal axons have remained viable [39]. In the case of a nerve injury with substantial nerve loss between the proximal and distal stump the gap would have to be bridged with a living nerve graft. This can be done with either a vascularized living nerve autograft or with a tissue-engineered nerve graft with living nerve axons grown in the laboratory [20, 40].

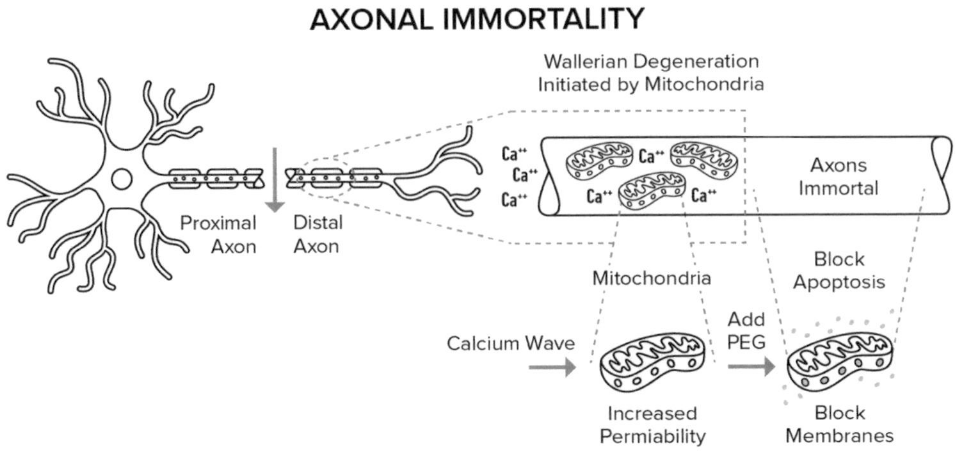


**Figure 3.**
*Axonal Immortality (Section 2.3). Distal axons in the distal stump undergo Wallerian degeneration after the injury of the peripheral nerve, either by the mechanism of being cut or crushed. There is also proximal degeneration (retrograde degeneration), similar to Wallerian degeneration, which involves several nodes of Ranvier proximal to the injury site. It is believed that a calcium wave causes increased permeability in the outer membrane of mitochondria in the axon, and this increased permeability allows bioagents such as enzymes to be released by the mitochondria. The increased permeability then initiates Wallerian degeneration by signaling the cascade that causes the Schwann cells to begin the process, recruit monocytes, and transform them into macrophages to remove the debris in the distal axons. If polyethylene glycol is released at the injury site it plugs the pores in the mitochondria and therefore blocks this Wallerian degeneration cascade. This leads to the axons becoming "immortal".*

Once we can keep the distal nerve stump alive along with its axons and Schwann cells, we will open up many possibilities for the future of brachial plexus surgery for acute injuries. What about chronic nerve injuries? We will address these in the next sections, for cases in which the upper limb has lost all of its function, the distal end organs of muscle have atrophied, the joints have become stiff and immobile, and even the distal nerve Schwann cells have undergone regression so there is no longer a distal nerve stump available for reconstruction to connect to the end-organs.

### *2.3.1 Preventing neuronal loss proximal to brachial plexus injuries*

It has been known for many decades that even distal nerve injuries result in the death of at least sensory neurons in the dorsal horn cells, and that more proximal injuries result in a very notable loss of motor neurons as well. Many feel that this loss of both sensory and motor neurons is responsible to a major degree for the observed poor outcomes following brachial plexus reconstruction. A living neuron can generate a new axon, but neurons cannot replicate themselves to repopulate neurons lost following peripheral nerve injuries. Some studies have shown that almost 80 percent of motor neurons die following nerve root avulsion, a frequent component of brachial plexus injuries in babies and adults. Such studies have shown that early repair has a protective mechanism whose etiology is not yet clear [41].

Such early repair observations have led researchers (i) to study the potential mechanisms associated with proximal neuronal apoptosis and by understanding the mechanisms, (ii) to seek to discover therapies to prevent proximal neuronal apoptosis. Recently investigators have found that N-Acetylcysteine prevents retrograde motor neuron death after neonatal peripheral nerve injury [42].

Other investigators found that altering transmembrane proteins that are selectively expressed on neurons and oligodendrocytes facilitated neuron survival and axonal regeneration, attenuated muscle atrophy and motor end-plate loss, enhanced neovascularization, and promoted functional recovery in a rat model [43].

As previously mentioned, mitochondrial dysfunction may play a role in neuronal apoptosis and mechanisms to reduce this role may be beneficial in preventing neuronal apoptosis. Over the coming years, we can easily anticipate the discovery of molecular solutions to proximal apoptosis along with novel delivery systems such as viral vectors.

## 3. Part II: Chronic injuries and treatment

### 3.1 Robotic limbs and brain-machine interfaces: Microelectronic axon processor

In the case of the most severe chronic brachial plexus injuries, the upper limb has become insensible and irreversibly paralyzed. The muscle end organs have atrophied. The neuromuscular junctions have resorbed. The distal nerve stump and its Schwann cells have regressed. There is no possibility to re-establish connectivity and conduction. In these most severe injuries, all of the roots of the brachial plexus have been avulsed. For these chronic patients, there is little to be gained by using nerve grafts from the contralateral seventh nerve root or other available donor nerve such as intercostals and the spinal accessory nerve to innervate the very few functional muscles that can be transferred from other parts of the body, such as the lower limbs. In these cases, the patient's surgical options for limb repair are severely limited. Often if they have one normal upper limb, they may opt not to proceed with a reconstruction of the functionless limb. One alternative is to consider amputation and replacement of the absent limb with an artificial prosthetic limb. There have been great strides made in robotic limbs in the past two decades [44]. Researchers have created endoskeletons; artificial or robotic prostheses that replace an entire amputated arm. There has also been significant progress in restoring function with an exoskeleton – a robotic device that is attached to the outside of the paralyzed limb, allowing it to move and in some cases have sensory function. For both the endoskeleton and exoskeleton prosthetics, phenomenal progress has been made in macrorobotics and microrobotics to enable the fabrication of limbs with dexterity that approaches the human upper limb.

New lightweight materials with increased strength have been used employing new fabrication techniques. These fabrication approaches include new computer-controlled milling machines and machines that extrude materials layer-by-layer at micrometer scale to build a full arm. These design and fabrication approaches allow us to now match the properties of a bird's wing skeleton with respect to both increased strength and decreased weight. Projects both in the US and globally have made huge strides in their production of robotic limbs. One project proposed a brain-machine interface (BMI) to control the new arms that would enable a direct coupling of signals from the brain to control the micromotors powering the new artificial limbs (**Figure 4**). This was pioneered by a number of universities. Even as the BMIs improved, many artificial arms continue to be controlled by more conventional myoelectric systems that use electrical impulses from surface electrodes placed over muscles not involved in the brachial plexus injury. In other cases, increased functional connections have been made in muscle units by dividing muscles into smaller segments and instrumenting these smaller units to control more degrees of freedom available in the robotic limbs.

BMIs have become ever more sophisticated with implants of specialized electrodes into the brain and in some cases, biological interfaces [20, 40, 45].

Work at Stanford by one of the authors envisioned a microelectonic axon processer (MAP) to interface with available peripheral nerves. The MAP would be coupled

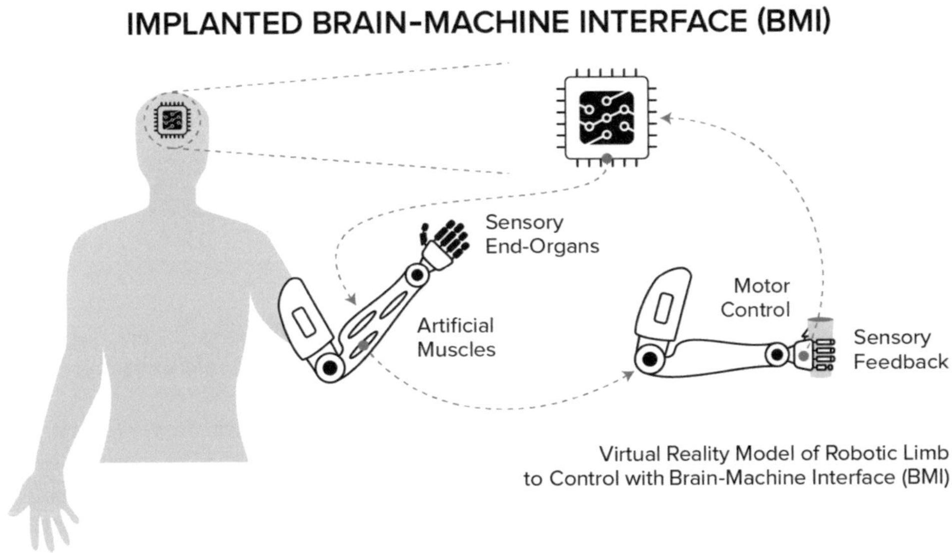


**Figure 4.**
*Virtual Reality Model of a Robotic Limb Controlled by Brain-Machine Interfaces (BMIs) (Section 3.1). Robotic prostheses can serve as replacements for the missing limb, or as exoskeletons attached to the surface of the flail limb to replace the loss of limb function after a chronic severe avulsion injury of the pan brachial plexus. The robotic limb can be controlled with surface electrodes or be directly coupled to computer chips or deep brain electrodes placed in the brain or on the surface of the brain like an electroencephalogram (EEG). Deep brain stimulus is already widely used clinically. In this case, similar electrodes would be used to either (1) provide motor commands or inputs from the brain to the robotic limb or exoskeleton, or (2) provide sensory feedback from the limb to the brain.*

to a peripheral nerve at a repair site and the proximal axons would connect to the distal axons through micrometer holes. Each hole would be instrumented with a recording and stimulator electrode as part of a dynamic random access memory (DRAM) microelectronic chip. The electrode sites would be made of iridium on iridium contacts that would improve the signal to noise ratio and would help to prevent the formation of scar tissue at the interface from causing decrements in the signal quality. Although this work was begun in the 1980s it was very much ahead of its time, as there is no present device with the same function.

Laboratory models of these chips were successfully tested in animal models. The thousands of electrode sites mounted on the chip could then be programmed using mirror technology programs taking advantage of artificial intelligence algorithms using neural networks. This would allow the nerves to communicate in a bidirectional manner with the robotic limbs at an axon level providing true detailed connections of the motor and sensory systems at the level of the full maximum set of degrees of freedom presently available in the human upper extremity.

First, we will see the introduction of simple BMIs but over time, we will see more and more complex BMIs to control the robotic limbs whether they are a full replacement of a limb or an exoskeleton fitted seamlessly around the non-functional human limb.

### *3.1.1 Robotic limbs and brain-machine interfaces (additional reading)*

In these additional readings, one can learn more about upper limb prosthetics [46] including an advanced prosthetic called the DEKA arm [47, 48] and other advances funded by defense advanced research projects agency (DARPA), [49] interfaces involved in control of prosthetics, [50–54] exoskeletons, [55] and considerations for different levels of amputation [56].

| Reference | Topic overview |
|---|---|
| [46] | A review including technological advances in prosthetics for upper limb amputees |
| [47] | A case series studying the DEKA arm– a prosthetic upper limb with active wrist control |
| [48] | An article exploring the various DEKA arm models created through funding from DARPA |
| [49] | A review discussing DARPA-funded peripheral nerve interfaces including a focus on provision of motor control and sensory feedback to prosthetic limbs |
| [50] | A review summarizing biosignal processing of BMIs that utilize EEG and EMG signals, as well as a discussion of sensors, features, and classifiers for upper limb prosthetics |
| [51] | A review investigating the impact of biomechatronic technology on amputee rehabilitation outcomes, including upper limb amputees |
| [52] | This book chapter discusses the way electromyography (EMG) is used to create pattern-based myoelectric movements of upper limb prosthetics |
| [53] | A clinical trial studying the use of Utah Slanted Electrode Arrays (USEAs) to provide more degrees of freedom in movement and increased proprioception for prosthetic hand users |
| [54] | A review of the state-of-the-art and the limitations of myoelectric signal control methods of upper limb prostheses |
| [55] | A systematic review of EEG used in BMIs for control of human limb exoskeletons, including background on upper limb exoskeletons |
| [56] | A review exploring exoprosthetic limb replacement considering different severities of amputation to the upper limb |

### 3.2 Genetic engineering, growing new limbs, and transplantation of limbs

Many brachial plexus patients will refuse an amputation of their chronically denervated atrophied stiff limb. In these cases, it should be possible to take advantage of the advances in allotransplantation. The first kidney transplantation was performed 70 years ago and vital life-saving organ transplantation has become a major contribution to our surgical armamentarium for hearts, lungs, kidneys, livers, and other parts. We have seen a more recent increase in the allotransplantion of both faces and limbs. Hand transplants have become an everyday reality. They could also be used to replace non-functional limbs in combination with new approaches to keep the distal segment of the peripheral nerve functional to allow immediate reconnection of the nerves of the transplanted limb to the proximal stumps of the brachial plexus through the use of fusogens. However, two key limitations remain: the supply of donor-appropriate limbs and controlling the immune system [57]. Improvements in immune suppression have helped to overcome rejection and reduced the associated risks of immune suppression [58]. Research in modulating the immune system continues to result in major strides both for solid organs and allotransplantation of faces and limbs. However, the ultimate future solution for the limited supply of donor parts will be the ability to use either (i) regenerative medicine to grow a new limb or (ii) genetic engineering with new tools such as CRISPR to change our genetic code to let humans do what many other creatures can do – regenerate a totally new limb from an amputated stump. Limb regeneration will require breakthroughs that are beyond the timeframe of this chapter, and it will fall to others to speculate about the future beyond the next 40 years. For now, we are limited to transplanted limbs and the inherent limitations of immune suppression and supply of donor limbs.

#### *3.2.1 Genetic engineering, limb growth, and transplantation (additional reading)*

These additional readings further describe hand transplant background [59] and outcomes, [59, 60] immunosuppression needed for vascularized composite allotransplantation (VCA), [61, 62] complications in VCA, [63] and transplant waiting lists [64].

| Reference | Topic overview |
|---|---|
| [59] | A review paper including hand transplant background and outcomes |
| [60] | A review of hand and upper extremity transplantation outcomes |
| [61] | A review of immunosuppression in VCA including approaches and future directions |
| [62] | A review discussing outcomes, resultant functionality, and immunosuppression in VCA procedures. |
| [63] | A review summarizing complications that have occurred in VCA |
| [64] | A review exploring the VCA waiting list in the US |

### 3.3 Computers, virtual reality, augmented reality, and artificial intelligence

Computers were a product of World War II and there has been exponential progression over the past 75 years. The microprocessors powering computers have followed Moore's law, doubling their computational ability every two years for the past 40 years. This will eventually enable the development of a microelectronic axon processor as we have discussed above in Section 3.1. Computers and their computational power will let us design truly realistic models of the brachial plexus injuries facing us in the operating room. Mathematical models can mimic the behavior of the nervous tissue and other surgical tissues that we need to manipulate. These models will enable a future surgeon to visualize the brachial plexus and a specific injury in real time in a virtual reality environment. It can now be used to train surgeons and to prepare, plan, and practice surgeries prior to attempting to repair the most complex brachial plexus injuries. A virtual reality helmet or viewer such as the Oculus™ can link to a computer model of a specific injury, created using a physically-based finite element mathematical model of the brachial plexus and surrounding tissues of a patient, from data obtained from a detail-rich 3D MRI, CT scan, or ultrasound taken prior to surgery. Surgical simulation has now become an accepted tool in many of our fields since its inception in the 1980s. The original applications modeled gunshot ballistic injuries and congenital problems such as surgery on cerebral palsy. Once virtual reality established the use for these models for planning and practicing surgery, then it became possible to apply the same patient-specific models in the operating room by superimposing the models on the patient as we operated (on the patient – a technology known as augmented reality **Figure 5**). There exist several systems that enable the fusion of the computer-based mathematical model of the patient that was created prior to the surgery onto the actual patient during the procedure. The term coined for this by one of the authors is a "performance machine."

A performance machine allows the surgeon to conduct the surgery with the aid of the computer model and ultimately to predict the outcomes. The most advanced models with the aid of artificial intelligence will predict the outcomes of surgery. Outcome prediction has been done [65] in other fields such as musculoskeletal surgery and vascular surgery, and should eventually be possible for peripheral nerve surgery such as complex brachial plexus surgery. Although computationally intense, it is possible to accurately fuse the computer model on the actual patient in real time as we are performing the surgery. With the overlay of the computer model, we can "see through" the tissue that surrounds the brachial plexus, identify key landmarks, and avoid key structures. Surgeons also often use the surgical robot in performing brachial plexus surgery in areas that are difficult to reach, for example, beneath the clavicle in the area of the subclavian vessels. Our most challenging cases are in brachial plexus surgery or injuries where the subclavian vessels have been repaired or bypassed, and the normal surgical planes have become obliterated by scar.
In a similar manner where a tumor may encircle the brachial plexus, combining

computer simulation and robotic surgery technologies (**Figure 6**) may reduce some of the risks inherent in such cases. Each year we come closer to seeing virtual and augmented reality technologies introduced in brachial plexus surgery.

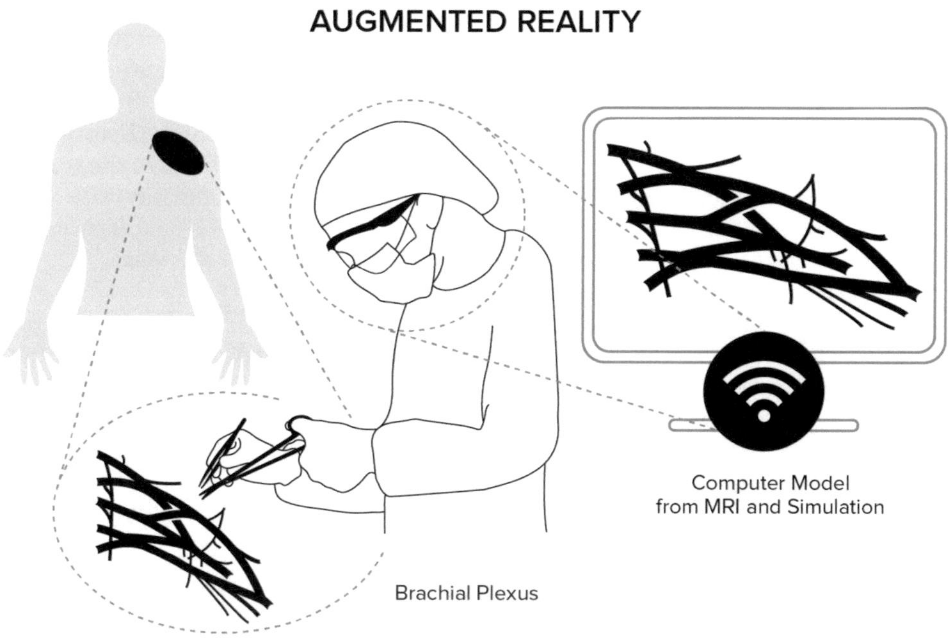


**Figure 5.**
*Augmented Reality (Section 3.3). In augmented reality, we create 3D image models of the brachial plexus for a specific patient and then superimpose these images on the patient's body in real time during the surgical procedure. This superimposed 3D model allows the surgeon to "see into" the patient as the model displays transparent skin, soft tissue and bones to pinpoint the exact position of the nerves. The model can deform and change shape, adjust to the position of the patient and the brachial plexus with the patient location using fiducials or key markers that allow the computer the fuse the patient and the models together in the same space. These models can be combined with robotic surgery to allow the surgeon to use a minimally invasive approach to the brachial plexus, working around critical structures such as vessels and bones.*

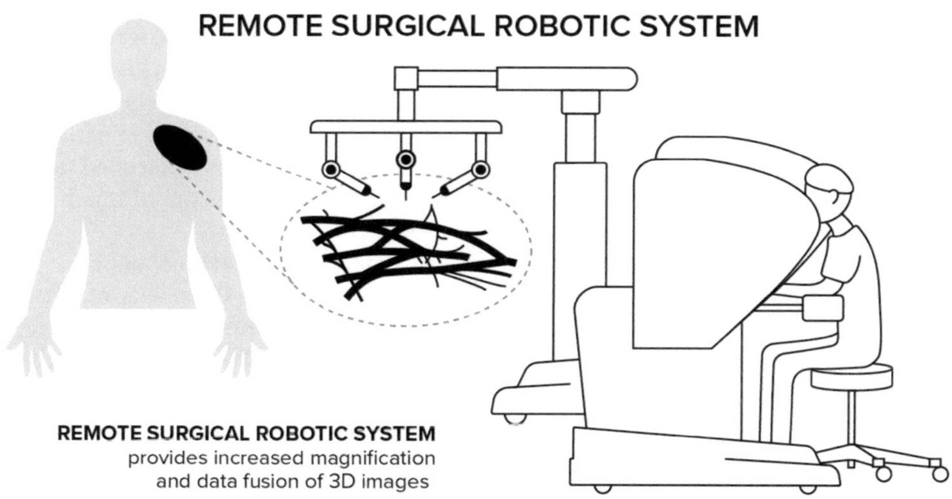


**Figure 6.**
*Robotics (Section 3.3). This remote surgical robotic system uses a surgical robot to assist the surgeon in operating on the brachial plexus. This system provides increased magnification, removes the surgeon's tremor, and provides the ability for data fusion of pre-acquired 3D images.*

Another promising development in computers is the use of artificial intelligence (AI) in decision-making. We have done research in modeling surgical cases to improve the communication between the patient, the physicians, and surgeons [66]. These models have used the AI discipline of Bayesian algorithms to model the behavior of the patient and the physician during complicated procedures [67]. Lack of communication or miscommunication can lead to poor outcomes where the needs of the patient and the decisions made by the surgeon are misaligned. It is possible to develop models based on AI that can help to reduce these errors [68]. Brachial plexus surgery is an especially rich area for this type of decision-making because of the complexity of the decision-making and the many choices available to the surgical team in deciding which is the best course of action for the patient [66, 69, 70].

### *3.3.1 Virtual reality, augmented reality, and artificial intelligence (additional reading)*

One can learn about virtual reality, augmented reality and artificial intelligence by reading about models that capture decision-making processes, [71] Bayesian 2-test cases in medicine, [72] and VR and AR use in medical imaging [73] and procedures [74].

| Reference | Topic overview |
|---|---|
| [71] | A proceeding that utilized a cognitive model to capture decision-making processes |
| [72] | An article exploring the use of visual aids to better demonstrate results of Bayesian 2-test cases in the medical field |
| [73] | A review investigating the use of VR and AR in medical image viewing/manipulation, including background on VR and AR development |
| [74] | A review exploring the documented uses of VR and AR in medicine, including in diagnostic and surgical procedures |

## 4. Conclusion: brave new world of brachial plexus surgery

In looking forward, as Sir Isaac Newton was quoted as saying in 1695, "If I have seen further than others, it is by standing on the shoulders of giants."[2] Many scientists and clinicians have provided the foundation that we presently stand upon. The authors have contributed to many of these fields, but many others have led these fields and created the technologies that we discussed in this chapter that can, one day, further advance the field of brachial plexus surgery. This chapter cannot possibly give credit to all of those scientists and clinicians that have preceded us. However, our goal has been to look at possible scenarios for the future of brachial plexus surgery and provide an optimistic view of the future.

This optimistic view sees a future in which a patient with a severe brachial plexus injury can dream of, hope for and ultimately experience the reality of a fully functional limb, whether biological or artificial, following their treatment. The solutions in the future will stem from many of the present technologies and methodologies that we have presented in this chapter. But these are only our vision for

[2] "If I have seen further," Isaac Newton wrote in a 1675 letter to fellow scientist Robert Hooke, "it is by standing on the shoulders of giants." https://fs.blog/2020/04/shoulders-of-giants/. This was a saying that was well known in Newton's time and he was paraphraing it: (https://www.quora.com/When-Newton-said-If-I-have-seen-further-it-is-because-I-have-stood-on-the-shoulders-of-giants-to-whom-was-he-referring-Who-were-his-giants).

the future. We are sure that there are other technologies that we have not discussed, and ones that we have not foreseen, that will impact this field.

During our careers our most severe challenges have been seeing our unfortunate patients with brachial plexus injuries that do not turn out well, whether a child with a birth defect, or an adult with a traumatic injury. They have been among our most courageous and most thankful patients. It is important that we dedicate ourselves through our careers to help them in any way that we can. We will participate in many successes and failures as we introduce new technologies and surgical techniques to address the many challenges presented by this field. It is through our patients and our camaraderie to share our knowledge, our successes and our failures, that we will move this field forward. This book is an important milestone in our field and we feel fortunate to have contributed this chapter to the success of this book. Its publication is very timely to mark the past progress in this field, the present state of the field, and in some small part, to look at the future ahead of us as practitioners of the field of brachial plexus surgery.

## Acknowledgements

The authors wish to acknowledge Robyn Mosher, MS, for manuscript editing, literature searches, and reference management; and Linnea Spelman, BA, for image design and production, editing, and proofreading.

## Author details

Joseph M. Rosen[1,2*], Jennifer Hong[3], Julien Klaudt-Moreau[4], Allison Podsednik[4] and Vincent R. Hentz[5]

1 Professor of Surgery and Engineering, Dartmouth-Hitchcock Medical Center, Lebanon NH, USA

2 Thayer School of Engineering, Hanover, NH, USA

3 Assistant Professor of Surgery and of Molecular and Systems Biology, Departments of Surgery and Molecular and Systems Biology, (Peripheral Nerve Surgery Specialist), Dartmouth-Hitchcock Medical Center, Lebanon, NH, USA

4 Clinical Research Assistant, Thayer School of Engineering at Dartmouth, Hanover, NH, USA

5 Emeritus Professor of Surgery, Stanford Medical Center, Stanford, CA, USA

*Address all correspondence to: joseph.m.rosen@gmail.com

## References


[1] Kovacs GT, Storment CW, Rosen JM. Regeneration microelectrode array for peripheral nerve recording and stimulation. IEEE Trans Biomed Eng. 1992;39(9):893-902.

[2] Jiang L, Jones S, Jia X. Stem cell transplantation for peripheral nerve regeneration: current options and opportunities. Int J Mol Sci. 2017;18(1).

[3] Gu X, Ding F, Williams DF. Neural tissue engineering options for peripheral nerve regeneration. Biomaterials. 2014;35(24):6143-56.

[4] Katiyar KS, Burrell JC, Laimo FA, Browne KD, Bianchi JR, Walters A, et al. Biomanufacturing of axon-based tissue engineered nerve grafts using porcine galsafe neurons. Tissue Eng Part A. 2021.

[5] Katiyar KS, Struzyna LA, Morand JP, Burrell JC, Clements B, Laimo FA, et al. Tissue engineered axon tracts serve as living scaffolds to accelerate axonal regeneration and functional recovery following peripheral nerve injury in rats. Front Bioeng Biotechnol. 2020;8:492.

[6] Yokoi T, Uemura T, Takamatsu K, Onode E, Shintani K, Hama S, et al. Long-term survival of transplanted induced pluripotent stem cell-derived neurospheres with nerve conduit into sciatic nerve defects in immunosuppressed mice. Biochem Biophys Rep. 2021;26:100979.

[7] Mathot F, Rbia N, Thaler R, Bishop AT, van Wijnen AJ, Shin AY. Introducing human adipose-derived mesenchymal stem cells to Avance ® nerve grafts and NeuraGen ® nerve guides. J Plast Reconstr Aesthet Surg. 2020;73(8):1473-81.

[8] Yin Y, Xiao G, Zhang K, Ying G, Xu H, De Melo BAG, et al. Tacrolimus — and nerve growth factor — treated allografts for neural tissue regeneration. ACS Chem Neurosci. 2019;10(3):1411-9.

[9] Wang B, Huang M, Shang D, Yan X, Zhao B, Zhang X. Mitochondrial behavior in axon degeneration and regeneration. Front Aging Neurosci. 2021;13:650038.

[10] Liu D, Mi D, Zhang T, Zhang Y, Yan J, Wang Y, et al. Tubulation repair mitigates misdirection of regenerating motor axons across a sciatic nerve gap in rats. Sci Rep. 2018;8(1):3443.

[11] Kubiak CA, Kung TA, Brown DL, Cederna PS, Kemp SWP. State-of-the-art techniques in treating peripheral nerve injury. Plast Reconstr Surg. 2018;141(3):702-10.

[12] Jia H, Wang Y, Chen J, Li JP, Han HQ, Tong XJ, et al. Combination of BMSCs-laden acellular nerve xenografts transplantation and G-CSF administration promotes sciatic nerve regeneration. Synapse. 2019;73(7): e22093.

[13] Piovesana R, Faroni A, Tata AM, Reid AJ. Schwann-like adipose-derived stem cells as a promising therapeutic tool for peripheral nerve regeneration: effects of cholinergic stimulation. Neural Regen Res. 2021;16(6):1218-20.

[14] Wu SH, Liao YT, Hsueh KK, Huang HK, Chen TM, Chiang ER, et al. Adipose-derived mesenchymal stem cells from a hypoxic culture improve neuronal differentiation and nerve repair. Front Cell Dev Biol. 2021;9:658099.

[15] Zhang RC, Du WQ, Zhang JY, Yu SX, Lu FZ, Ding HM, et al. Mesenchymal stem cell treatment for peripheral nerve injury: a narrative review. Neural Regen Res. 2021;16(11): 2170-6.

[16] Kubiak CA, Grochmal J, Kung TA, Cederna PS, Midha R, Kemp SWP. Stem-cell-based therapies to enhance peripheral nerve regeneration. Muscle Nerve. 2020;61(4):449-59.

[17] Lavorato A, Raimondo S, Boido M, Muratori L, Durante G, Cofano F, et al. Mesenchymal stem cell treatment perspectives in peripheral nerve regeneration: systematic review. Int J Mol Sci. 2021;22(2).

[18] Yin K, Divakar P, Hong J, Moodie KL, Rosen JM, Sundback CA, et al. Freeze-cast porous chitosan conduit for peripheral nerve repair. MRS Adv. 2018;3(30):1677-83.

[19] Wieringa PA, Goncalves de Pinho AR, Micera S, van Wezel RJA, Moroni L. Biomimetic architectures for peripheral nerve repair: a review of biofabrication strategies. Adv Healthc Mater. 2018;7(8):e1701164.

[20] Maggiore JC, Burrell JC, Browne KD, Katiyar KS, Laimo FA, Ali ZS, et al. Tissue engineered axon-based "living scaffolds" promote survival of spinal cord motor neurons following peripheral nerve repair. J Tissue Eng Regen Med. 2020;14(12): 1892-907.

[21] Patel NP, Lyon KA, Huang JH. An update-tissue engineered nerve grafts for the repair of peripheral nerve injuries. Neural Regen Res. 2018;13(5):764-74.

[22] Kennedy KM, Bhaw-Luximon A, Jhurry D. Cell-matrix mechanical interaction in electrospun polymeric scaffolds for tissue engineering: Implications for scaffold design and performance. Acta Biomater. 2017;50:41-55.

[23] Neumann B, Linton C, Giordano-Santini R, Hilliard MA. Axonal fusion: An alternative and efficient mechanism of nerve repair. Prog Neurobiol. 2019;173:88-101.

[24] Ye Y, Kim CY, Miao Q, Ren X. Fusogen-assisted rapid reconstitution of anatomophysiologic continuity of the transected spinal cord. Surgery. 2016;160(1):20-5.

[25] Bittner GD, Sengelaub DR, Trevino RC, Peduzzi JD, Mikesh M, Ghergherehchi CL, et al. The curious ability of polyethylene glycol fusion technologies to restore lost behaviors after nerve severance. J Neurosci Res. 2016;94(3):207-30.

[26] Abdou SA, Henderson PW. Fusogens: chemical agents that can rapidly restore function after nerve injury. J Surg Res. 2019;233:36-40.

[27] Vargas SA, Bittner GD. Natural mechanisms and artificial PEG-induced mechanism that repair traumatic damage to the plasmalemma in eukaryotes. Curr Top Membr. 2019;84:129-67.

[28] Riley DC, Boyer RB, Deister CA, Pollins AC, Cardwell NL, Kelm ND, et al. Immediate enhancement of nerve function using a novel axonal fusion device after neurotmesis. Ann Plast Surg. 2017;79(6):590-9.

[29] Bamba R, Waitayawinyu T, Nookala R, Riley DC, Boyer RB, Sexton KW, et al. A novel therapy to promote axonal fusion in human digital nerves. J Trauma Acute Care Surg. 2016;81(5 Suppl 2 Proceedings of the 2015 Military Health System Research Symposium):S177-s83.

[30] Messineo E, Pollins A, Thayer W. Optimization and evaluation of an in vitro model of PEG-mediated fusion of nerve cell bodies. J Clin Neurosci. 2019;63:189-95.

[31] Baron A, Strohl A. Severe Cubital Tunnel Syndrome: considerations for nerve transfer surgery. Curr Rev Musculoskelet Med. 2020;13(6):708-16.

[32] Sullivan R, Dailey T, Duncan K, Abel N, Borlongan CV. Peripheral nerve injury: stem cell therapy and peripheral nerve transfer. Int J Mol Sci. 2016;17(12).

[33] Wells ME, Gonzalez GA, Childs BR, Williams MR, Nesti LJ, Dunn JC. Radial to axillary nerve transfer outcomes in shoulder abduction: a systematic review. Plast Reconstr Surg Glob Open. 2020;8(9):e3096.

[34] Hardcastle N, Texakalidis P, Nagarajan P, Tora MS, Boulis NM. Recovery of shoulder abduction in traumatic brachial plexus palsy: a systematic review and meta-analysis of nerve transfer versus nerve graft. Neurosurg Rev. 2020;43(3):951-6.

[35] Cheng XT, Sheng ZH. Developmental regulation of microtubule-based trafficking and anchoring of axonal mitochondria in health and diseases. Dev Neurobiol. 2021;81(3):284-99.

[36] Ghergherehchi CL, Bittner GD, Hastings RL, Mikesh M, Riley DC, Trevino RC, et al. Effects of extracellular calcium and surgical techniques on restoration of axonal continuity by polyethylene glycol fusion following complete cut or crush severance of rat sciatic nerves. J Neurosci Res. 2016;94(3):231-45.

[37] Ghergherehchi CL, Mikesh M, Sengelaub DR, Jackson DM, Smith T, Nguyen J, et al. Polyethylene glycol (PEG) and other bioactive solutions with neurorrhaphy for rapid and dramatic repair of peripheral nerve lesions by PEG-fusion. J Neurosci Methods. 2019;314:1-12.

[38] Bittner GD, Sengelaub DR, Ghergherehchi CL. Conundrums and confusions regarding how polyethylene glycol-fusion produces excellent behavioral recovery after peripheral nerve injuries. Neural Regen Res. 2018;13(1):53-7.

[39] Paskal AM, Paskal W, Pietruski P, Wlodarski PK. Polyethylene glycol: the future of posttraumatic nerve repair? Systemic review. Int J Mol Sci. 2019;20(6).

[40] Burrell JC, Browne KD, Dutton JL, Laimo FA, Das S, Brown DP, et al. A porcine model of peripheral nerve injury enabling ultra-long regenerative distances: surgical approach, recovery kinetics, and clinical relevance. Neurosurgery. 2020;87(4):833-46.

[41] Bourke G, McGrath AM, Wiberg M, Novikov LN. Effects of early nerve repair on experimental brachial plexus injury in neonatal rats. J Hand Surg Eur Vol. 2018;43(3):275-81.

[42] Catapano J, Zhang J, Scholl D, Chiang C, Gordon T, Borschel GH. N-Acetylcysteine prevents retrograde motor neuron death after neonatal peripheral nerve injury. Plast Reconstr Surg. 2017;139(5):1105e-15e.

[43] Ding L, Zhu Z, Wang Y, Zeng L, Wang T, Luo J, et al. LINGO-1 shRNA Loaded by Pluronic F-127 Promotes Functional Recovery After Ventral Root Avulsion. Tissue Eng Part A. 2019;25(19-20):1381-95.

[44] Kubiak CA, Etra JW, Brandacher G, Kemp SWP, Kung TA, Lee WPA, et al. Prosthetic rehabilitation and vascularized composite allotransplantation following upper limb loss. Plast Reconstr Surg. 2019;143(6):1688-701.

[45] Miranda RA, Casebeer WD, Hein AM, Judy JW, Krotkov EP, Laabs TL, et al. DARPA-funded efforts in the development of novel brain-computer interface technologies. J Neurosci Methods. 2015;244:52-67.

[46] Geary M, Gaston RG, Loeffler B. Surgical and technological advances in the management of upper limb amputees. Bone Joint J. 2021;103-B(3): 430-9.

[47] Cowley J, Resnik L, Wilken J, Smurr Walters L, Gates D. Movement quality of conventional prostheses and the DEKA Arm during everyday tasks. Prosthet Orthot Int. 2017;41(1):33-40.

[48] Resnik L, Klinger SL, Etter K. The DEKA Arm: its features, functionality, and evolution during the Veterans Affairs Study to optimize the DEKA Arm. Prosthet Orthot Int. 2014;38(6):492-504.

[49] Naufel S, Knaack GL, Miranda R, Best TK, Fitzpatrick K, Emondi AA, et al. DARPA investment in peripheral nerve interfaces for prosthetics, prescriptions, and plasticity. J Neurosci Methods. 2020;332:108539.

[50] Khan SM, Khan AA, Farooq O. Selection of features and classifiers for EMG-EEG-based upper limb assistive devices-a review. IEEE Rev Biomed Eng. 2020;13:248-60.

[51] Lechler K, Frossard B, Whelan L, Langlois D, Muller R, Kristjansson K. Motorized biomechatronic upper and lower limb prostheses-clinically relevant outcomes. PM R. 2018;10(9 Suppl 2):S207-S19.

[52] Li G, Samuel OW, Lin C, Asogbon MG, Fang P, Idowu PO. Realizing efficient emg-based prosthetic control strategy. Adv Exp Med Biol. 2019;1101:149-66.

[53] Wendelken S, Page DM, Davis T, Wark HAC, Kluger DT, Duncan C, et al. Restoration of motor control and proprioceptive and cutaneous sensation in humans with prior upper-limb amputation via multiple Utah Slanted Electrode Arrays (USEAs) implanted in residual peripheral arm nerves. J Neuroeng Rehabil. 2017;14(1):121.

[54] Yang D, Gu Y, Thakor NV, Liu H. Improving the functionality, robustness, and adaptability of myoelectric control for dexterous motion restoration. Exp Brain Res. 2019;237(2):291-311.

[55] Al-Quraishi MS, Elamvazuthi I, Daud SA, Parasuraman S, Borboni A. EEG-based control for upper and lower limb exoskeletons and prostheses: a systematic review. Sensors (Basel). 2018;18(10).

[56] Salminger S, Mayer JA, Sturma A, Riedl O, Bergmeister KD, Aszmann OC. [Article in German]. Z Orthop Unfall. 2016;154(4):411-24.

[57] Benedict J, Magill G. Upper extremity and craniofacial vascularized composite allotransplantation: ethics and immunosuppression. Emerg Top Life Sci. 2019;3(6):681-6.

[58] Kollar B, Pomahac B, Riella LV. Novel immunological and clinical insights in vascularized composite allotransplantation. Curr Opin Organ Transplant. 2019;24(1):42-8.

[59] Carlsen BT, Prigge P, Peterson J. Upper extremity limb loss: functional restoration from prosthesis and targeted reinnervation to transplantation. J Hand Ther. 2014;27(2):106-13; quiz 114.

[60] Shores JT, Brandacher G, Lee WPA. Hand and upper extremity transplantation: an update of outcomes in the worldwide experience. Plast Reconstr Surg. 2015;135(2):351e-60e.

[61] Kueckelhaus M, Fischer S, Seyda M, Bueno EM, Aycart MA, Alhefzi M, et al. Vascularized composite allotransplantation: current standards and novel approaches to prevent acute rejection and chronic allograft deterioration. Transpl Int. 2016;29(6):655-62.

[62] Shores JT, Malek V, Lee WPA, Brandacher G. Outcomes after hand and upper extremity transplantation. J Mater Sci Mater Med. 2017;28(5):72.

[63] Uluer MC, Brazio PS, Woodall JD, Nam AJ, Bartlett ST, Barth RN. Vascularized composite allotransplantation: medical complications. Curr Transplant Rep. 2016;3(4):395-403.

[64] Wainright JL, Wholley CL, Cherikh WS, Musick JM, Klassen DK. OPTN vascularized composite allograft waiting list: current status and trends in the United States. Transplantation. 2018;102(11):1885-90.

[65] Elfanagely O, Toyoda Y, Othman S, Mellia JA, Basta M, Liu T, et al. Machine learning and surgical outcomes prediction: a systematic review. J Surg Res. 2021;264:346-61.

[66] Santos Jr. E, Rosen J, Kim K, Li D, Yu F, Guo Y, et al. Reasoning about intentions in complex organizational behavior. In: Salas E, Fiore S, Letsky M, editors. Theories of team cognition: cross-disciplinary perspectives Routledge: Taylor & Francis Group; 2011.

[67] Kyrimi E, Dube K, Fenton N, Fahmi A, Neves MR, Marsh W, et al. Bayesian networks in healthcare: What is preventing their adoption? Artif Intell Med. 2021;116:102079.

[68] Manski CF. Reasonable patient care under uncertainty. Health Econ. 2018;27(10):1397-421.

[69] Santos Jr. E, Rosen J, Kim KJ, Yu F, Li D, Jacob E, et al. Promoting Team Performance in the Operating room by analyzing gaps among surgical care members. In: Sokolowski JA, Banks CM, editors. Modeling and Simulation in the Medical and Health Sciences: Wiley, Inc.; 2010.

[70] Santos Jr. E, Rosen J, Kim K, Yu F, Li D, Jacob E, et al. Patient care. In: Sokolowski JA, Banks CM, editors. Modeling and Simulation in the Medical and Health Sciences Wiley; 2011.

[71] Santos Jr. EN, H.; Russell, J.; Kim, K.; Veenhuis, L.; Boparai, R.; Stautland, T., editors. Capturing a commander's decision-making style. Proceedings of SPIE; 2017 May 5, 2017; Anaheim, California, US.

[72] Binder K, Krauss S, Bruckmaier G, Marienhagen J. Visualizing the Bayesian 2-test case: The effect of tree diagrams on medical decision making. PLoS One. 2018;13(3):e0195029.

[73] Sutherland J, Belec J, Sheikh A, Chepelev L, Althobaity W, Chow BJW, et al. Applying modern virtual and augmented reality technologies to medical images and models. J Digit Imaging. 2019;32(1):38-53.

[74] Yeung AWK, Tosevska A, Klager E, Eibensteiner F, Laxar D, Stoyanov J, et al. Virtual and augmented reality applications in medicine: analysis of the scientific literature. J Med Internet Res. 2021;23(2):e25499.